W9-AHU-208

what would mickey say?

To Governor & Mrs. Carcieri,
Enjoy The Journey &
keep swinging for The
fences!
Michael

what would mickey say?

Coaching Men to Health and Happiness

MICHAEL SAMUELSON

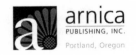

arnica
PUBLISHING, INC.
Portland, Oregon

Library of Congress Cataloging-in-Publication Data

Samuelson, Michael H.
   What would Mickey say? : coaching men to health and happiness / Michael
Samuelson.
      p. cm.
   Includes bibliographical references.
   ISBN 0-9726535-7-0 (pbk. : alk. paper)
   1. Men--Health and hygiene. 2. Men--Health and hygiene--Miscellanea. 3.
Happiness--Miscellanea. 4. Health. I. Title.

   RA777.8.S25 2004
   613'.04234--dc22

                                   2004007684

Copyright © 2005 by Michael Samuelson
All rights reserved.

This book may not be reproduced in whole or in part, by electronic or any
other means which exist or may yet be developed, without permission from:

Arnica Publishing
3739 SE 8th Avenue, Suite 1
Portland, OR 97202
www.arnicapublishing.com

Arnica books are available at special discounts when purchased in bulk for premiums and sales
promotions, as well as for fund-raising or educational use. Special editions or book excerpts can
also be created for specification. For details, contact the Sales Director at the address above.

This book is dedicated to men...and the women who love, nurture, encourage, guide, befriend, and tolerate us.

table of
contents

introduction

"Mantle swings...There goes a long drive...Going to deep right field...It's soaring up high, it's going, it's going, it is gone! A home run for Mickey Mantle and it almost went out of the ballpark. Mickey Mantle for the second time in his career has come within a few feet of becoming the first man to hit a ball out of Yankee Stadium!"

— MEL ALLEN, Yankee Stadium
May 30, 1956

The Mick did it again!
And it's my birthday!

The smile on my eight-year-old face lifts off the top of my head and sends ripples straight down to my toes. Reaching under my pillow, I turn down the volume wheel on my Arvin nine transistor radio and, as Mel Allen fades through the feathers, I close my eyes and once again hear the "Voice of the Yankees." *"Samuelson swings. There goes a long drive. It's soaring up high, it's going, it's going, it is gone! How about that, sports fans, the rookie is the first man to hit a ball out of Yankee Stadium!*

hero (n.) somebody who is admired and looked up to for outstanding qualities or achievements.

Mickey was it. The king. My idol. I copied his batting stance, tried to hit from both sides of the plate, played when hurt, and prided myself on the fact that, like Mickey, I was always swinging for the fences. Oh, there would be other baseball heroes like Roger Maris and Sandy Koufax, but nobody was even close to The Mick. He could do no wrong and I wanted to be just like him. As for other sports and players, they were just fillers until spring training called the Bronx Bombers back to Florida.

For other boys growing up in the fifties and early sixties, the heroes had names like Unitas, Howe, Palmer, Patterson, Russell, Andretti, Carter, and Gonzales. Generations before worshiped at the altars of Ruth, Lewis, Greenberg, Owens, DiMaggio, Thorpe, and Hogan. Kids growing up in the seventies and eighties chewed lots of bubble gum looking for Bench, Seaver, Namath, Orr, Byrd, or Magic. But in the summer of 1956, the blue, chipped plaster wall next to the bed on the second floor, front-right bedroom at 119 Hall Ave, Jamestown, New York had space for only one hero, Mickey Mantle.

Mickey's star brightened with the rocket growth of television in the late 1950s and early 1960s. The handsome, crew-cut, strong "ah-shucks" kind of a kid from Oklahoma who hit the ball a mile made a perfect Saturday matinee idol. When Dizzy Dean or Pee Wee Reese called him to the plate, flags waved and the scent of apple pie wafted throughout the house. You could even hear the sheets on the clothesline applaud as he stepped into the batter's box. Women thought he was cute, and guys wanted to be him. What Elvis was to rock 'n' roll, Mickey was to baseball.

He was a switch-hitting center fielder who played in 2,401 games for the New York Yankees from 1951 until 1968, won the Most Valuable Player award three times, hit a record eighteen homers in twelve World Series, and entered the Hall of Fame in 1974. In 1953 he slugged the longest home run ever measured, 565 ft., off Chuck Stobbs of the Washington Senators, and in 1956 he won the rare Triple Crown (.353 batting average, fifty-two homers, 130 runs batted in).

Those are the baseball facts. What us kids didn't know was how Mickey spent his time out of uniform.

Beginning at age nineteen, Mantle sprinted down a lifestyle road that would lead him to make this statement just weeks before his death: "God gave me everything and I blew it. For the kids out there, don't be like me!"

In his autobiography, *The Mick*, he writes: "If I tasted the high life in 1951, I got a bellyful starting in 1952—especially on the road. There were lots of parties, flashy people, hard liquor, and staying out really late. Billy [Martin] and I were often the life of the party. We wouldn't go upstairs to our old room until we were just about ready to drop." In *A Hero All of His Life: A Memoir by the Mantle Family,*

Mickey, his wife, Merlyn, and sons, Mickey Jr., David, and Danny, tell stories of verbal abuse to fans, alcoholism, life-long womanizing, and gut-wrenching regret.

Say it ain't so, Mick; say it ain't so!

THE PIN STRIPES WEAR THIN

For most of his career, Mickey Mantle lived under the protection of a no-tell press. Delighted with his Ruthian home runs, lightning speed, and rocket-arm, reporters shied away from his private life. The all-night carousing episodes with teammate buddies like Billy Martin, Whitey Ford, and Hank Bauer, legendary throughout the baseball world, stayed out of the papers (with one notable exception— a May 16, 1957 brawl at the Copacabana nightclub in New York City). However, the booze, philandering, and extended stays away from home took their toll on Mickey's health, marriage, and relationship with his sons. The out-of-control lifestyle would eventually destroy his liver, break up his marriage, and lead his boys down the path to alcoholism and periods of estrangement from their father. It would also take Mickey's life at the age of sixty-three.

LIVE, LOVE, AND BE MERRY BECAUSE TOMORROW...

A zinc miner's son raised in Commerce, Oklahoma, Mickey developed a fatalistic attitude about life and death as he watched first his grandfather then his father die of Hodgkin's disease. His father was only thirty-nine. Two uncles died of the same disease without living past their thirties. Believing this was his fate as well, he approached life with a reckless disregard for caution and a profound lack of common sense. He and Billy Martin used to joke about whose liver would give out first. Mickey won by default when Billy was killed in a one-car auto accident on Christmas Day, 1989.

Irony struck when the Hodgkin's disease Mantle expected to get himself skipped a generation and struck his son Billy (named after Billy Martin) when he was nineteen years old. Later, son Mickey, Jr. was also diagnosed with cancer. Billy died of a heart attack in 1994 at age thirty-six and Mickey, Jr. died of cancer in 2000 at the age of forty-seven.

After his baseball days were over in 1969, Mick made a living as a drinking buddy and golf partner for wealthy businessmen who wanted to tell their friends that they spent an afternoon with the great Mickey Mantle. When not on the golf course, he would often appear at baseball paraphernalia shows signing anything that fans put in front of him. Much of the time, however, he had nothing to do and no place to be.

Surprised to wake up forty-six years old and still breathing, he is often quoted as saying: "If I knew I was going to live this long, I would have taken better care of myself." In an article he did for *Sports Illustrated* in late 1993, he wrote, "It was when I had no commitments, nothing to do or nowhere to be that I lapsed into those long drinking sessions. It was the loneliness and emptiness. I found 'friends' at bars, and I filled my emptiness with alcohol." He described going through three or four bottles of wine in the course of an afternoon and needing six to eight vodka martinis before he could feel comfortable at a party. He often began his days with a drink he called "The Breakfast of Champions"—a big glass filled with a shot or more of brandy, some Kahlua, and cream. Tragically, though, he had little time for his sons while they were young, and when they grew up, he made them his drinking buddies.

In his later years, Mantle tried to correct his mistakes. He freely admitted his alcoholism, entered the Betty Ford Center, and made peace with his sons and his wife. Unfortunately, it was already too late.

Eighteen months into his new life of sobriety, the forty-two years of drinking caught up to him. On May 28, 1995, Mickey Mantle entered the Baylor Medical Center in Dallas, Texas complaining of stomach pains. A liver transplant followed—cancer had been discovered. Mantle died August 13 of liver cancer. He was sixty-three years old.

"It's what you learn after you know it all that counts."

— EARL WEAVER, Baseball Hall of Fame
Former Manager of the Baltimore Orioles

Mickey Mantle identified with the song *Yesterday When I Was Young*, made popular by Roy Clark, and asked that it be sung at his funeral.

So many wayward pleasures lay in store for me
And so much pain my dazzled eyes refused to see,
I ran so fast that time and youth at last ran out,
I never stopped to think what life was all about...
There are so many songs in me that won't be sung,
I feel the bitter taste of tears upon my tongue,
The time has come for me to pay for yesterday When I Was Young.

This curly-headed, eight-year-old from Jamestown, New York will always cherish the mythical Mickey—from the stickball alleys of the Bronx to the farm fields of Iowa, he brought hope, excitement, and fields of dreams to millions of baseball fans. He was as important to the developing American cultural landscape of the fifties and early sixties as Norman Rockwell, Ed Sullivan, Howdy Doodie, Kate Smith, Willie Mays, and Bob Hope. However, it is as an adult that I appreciate Mantle even more. Poetically fallible, he countered his on-field heroics with stumbles worthy of a Greek tragedy. And, in the echo of a familiar Biblical parable, he was, in the end, repentant and anxious to atone for his trespasses—he was our Prodigal Son.

In the sum of experience, which takes more courage and is the more heroic: to hit 536 home runs, or admit that you have squandered your life and talents while imploring kids not to follow in your footsteps?

Hey, Mick, the eight-year-old thanks you for the legend and this aging man who still dreams of "touchin' 'em all," thanks you for the lessons. You're still my hero.

"One of the beautiful things about baseball is that every once in awhile you come into a situation where you want to and where you have to reach down and prove something."

— NOLAN RYAN
Baseball Hall of Fame

Part of Mantle's legacy is this book, dedicated to men's health and happiness.

Using the informal setting of a company cafeteria, we will listen in on the conversations of everyday men as they talk about real-life issues—in their own words. Sex, relationships, alcohol, drugs, tobacco, sports, injuries, disease, career frustrations, exercise, aging, stress, work/life balance, spirituality, parenting, and food are discussed. And, just to keep the men honest, periodically, a woman or two stops by the lunch table for a chat.

Every day, in cafeterias all over the country, many different celebrities enter conversations as a way of driving home a point, filling time, or giving men an opening to obliquely share their personal lives. So is the case in our cafeteria. It may be a television star who risks everything for one more cocaine high, a politician who flaunts his marital infidelities, a rock star who commits suicide, or even a former president who continues to operate as if rules were meant only for others. They're all fair game at the lunch table.

COACH MANTLE

As the reader, you can simply sit back and eavesdrop for pure entertainment or you can add to the experience by reading the information captured in the two sections that close each chapter. One by one the lunchtime conversations touch subjects men talk about, including cancer, retirement, kids, women, and impotence (every guy's favorite…). As an example, we hear the men talk about what prostate cancer means (to them), listen to their fears, embarrassment, experiences, and, at times, misconceptions. Each chapter ends with two sections: What Would Mickey Say? and The Professor Speaks.

In the first section, Mickey Mantle, our lifestyle coach, demonstrates both down-to-earth, country-boy charm and reflective wisdom as he entertains and educates the reader with confessions, straight-talk, and do-not-do-as-I-did stories. In The Professor Speaks section, the reader is presented with research, fast facts, and professional recommendations related to that day's topics. In the ongoing spirit of fantasy, this clinical part of the book is presented by Professor Edwards from the local university.

DON'T BE LIKE ME…

It was at a press conference following his liver transplant surgery that Mantle told kids, "Don't be like me." At that same time, he looked straight ahead and said, "I'm going to spend the rest of my life trying to make it up."

When you read the loving account of his family in *A Hero All His Life,* there is no question that Mickey was sincere. Unfortunately, when he made this commitment he was up to bat in the bottom of the ninth in his most important game, and this time there was no dramatic, game-winning home run and the sheets did not applaud.

WHY THE WORKPLACE? AND, WHY A BOOK ON MEN'S HEALTH?

The answer to the first part of the question is easy—the second part takes a little longer.

Given that I am using Mickey Mantle as a lifestyle coach for men, why not make the setting a bar, a locker room, or, because he had an eleventh-hour conversion to Christianity, why not a place of worship? The primary reason for the workplace is because that is where men spend most of their time. Also, just as with The Mick, the dynamics of the home/work interactions have a tremendous impact on a man's health. A bad or good day at the office is the same regardless if your "office" is located on the assembly line at Ford Motor Company, in a penthouse suite on Fifth Ave., or center field at Yankee Stadium. Besides, the company cafeteria of a small (under 500-person) company gives me an opportunity to bring together men representing various social, cultural, economic, and educational backgrounds.

Why men?

The short answer is because, as men, we have done a miserable job of taking care of ourselves. For the longer answer, let's look at the facts.

According to The Men's Health Network—an excellent informational and educational organization located in Washington, D.C.—in 1920, the life expectancy gap between men and women was one year, but women in 2003 outlive men by seven years. Also, age-adjusted data indicate that the number of men who die from heart disease is double the number of women who die from heart disease and the incidence of stroke is 19 percent higher among men. Just as significant is the fact that 50 percent more men die of cancer than women and men are at least 25 percent less likely than women to visit a doctor.

"BOYS WILL BE BOYS" AND OTHER DANGEROUS NOTIONS

Of equal or greater concern is the fact that we are in a spiraling gender cycle of destruction that goes back for generations and shows no signs of breaking. At the extreme, it shows up in places like Paducah, Jonesboro, Cheyenne, Edinboro, and Columbine. Sociologists, psychologists, and anthropologists may debate over the amorphous origins of the masculinity mask (painted with toughness, stoicism, and bravado), but the results are concrete. As William Pollack reports in his superb work, *Real Boys*, boys are now twice as likely as girls to be labeled as "learning disabled," constitute up to 67 percent of our special education classes, and in some school systems are up to ten times more likely to be diagnosed with a serious emotional disorder— primarily attention deficit disorder (ADD). Also, while the significant gaps in girls' science and math achievement are improving greatly, boys' scores in reading are lagging behind significantly and continue to show little improvement. Recent studies also show that not only is a boy's self-esteem more fragile than that of a girl's and that boys' confidence as learners is impaired, but also that boys are substantially more likely to endure disciplinary problems, be suspended from classes, or actually drop out of school entirely.

As a one-time public school teacher and high school guidance counselor, I can report with vivid recall that this behavior and performance gap was present in the school systems back in the seventies and eighties, as well as today. In fact, it doesn't take a detailed study to convince anyone that this has been the case for as long as we can remember. Remember, "Boys will be boys...."

Of course, trouble for boys extends beyond the classroom walls and spills into everyday life. The rate of depression among today's boys is shockingly high and statistics now tell us that boys are up to three times more likely than girls to be the victims of a violent crime (other than sexual assault) and between four to six times more likely to commit suicide.

So, guys, it's time to take a diamond cutter's look at the damage we've done to the man (and boy) in the mirror—as well as the damage we've inflicted on others—and reflect on the importance of awareness and responsibility. And women, if you want to improve the quality of your lives and facilitate the creation and extension of quality years in the lives of your grandfathers, fathers, husbands, boyfriends, brothers, sons, and male friends, you have to start by paying closer attention to what the current system produces. To that end, I encourage you to lean close and listen to all the lunchroom discussions and commentary.

chapter
one

The Boy's Club
Meet the Guys

*W*e *begin with the narrator, Tom McGregor, introducing himself and providing some basic personal background. Tom is a recent addition to the company-sponsored softball team. The team is a diverse group of guys who are drawn together because of their love of the game. For five of the players, this bonding spread to the workplace cafeteria where they now sit at the same lunch table and comment on their personal lives, react to current events, muse, and just plain B.S.*

Although reluctant at first, the softball group now likes Tom enough to let him sit with them at their lunch table and, to borrow a basketball term, become the sixth man. Tom is pumped and is enjoying his new status as "one of the guys." More than simply sharing the table, we have a sense that Tom has earned their trust enough for them to talk freely about any topic—including work. Anxious to share what he is hearing and learning, Tom invites us (the readers) to gather around the table, listen to the guys, enjoy Mickey's commentary, and benefit from Professor Edwards' expertise.

The first chapter ends with a brief profile of each person at the table. The profiles provide basic personality information and foreshadow areas of potential concern. Each subsequent chapter highlights one or more of these concerns.

My name is Thomas Wesley McGregor—Tom. I am named, first, for my grandfather, and, second, for my mother's only brother.

I like to think of myself as a modern guy. I mean, I am not stuck in the old gender-typical world of my father or even my older brother for that matter. You know what I mean. The belief that men should be the primary breadwinners— women are the weaker sex—big boys don't cry—no pain, no gain, and similar ideas right out of *Gunsmoke*, *Superman*, *The Lone Ranger*, *Ozzie and Harriet*, *Leave It to Beaver*, and *The Brady Bunch*. Now, don't get me wrong, besides the obvious, I think there are other real differences between men and women. It's just that it's not that big of a deal. At least that's what I used to believe—until recently. Now, this far along in life, I'm not so sure.

ONCE UPON A TIME...

Before we go any further, let me give you some background:

The year I was born, 1948, Truman surprised just about everyone and was elected President of the United States, Gandhi was assassinated, Israel was declared an independent nation, Czechoslovakia was seized by the Soviet Union, Alfred Kinsey's book, *Sexual Behavior of the Human Male*, was published, a first-class stamp went for three cents, the Cleveland Indians won the World Series, and Babe Ruth died. If I were ten in 1948 instead of just a newborn, the only things to consciously touch my world would have been The Babe dying and the Yankees not playing baseball in October. The rest of it was for grown-ups.

I grew up in Jamestown, New York with a mom, a dad, two sisters, and two brothers. Stephen came first, then Dean, then me, and then, to my mother's great delight, the girls, Dorothy and Melissa. According to pop psychology, that makes me Thomas in the Middle—the forgotten one, although I never felt that way.

My dad and mom stayed together in a marriage that began when she was eighteen and he was twenty-one. Judging by old photo albums, the marriage flashed brightly at one time; however, I never saw the joy first-hand. Mostly, I remember my dad retreating to a warm bottle of beer pulled from a crinkled brown paper bag hidden on a ledge behind the second step leading down to the basement, and my mom counting the beads on her rosary. Dad's three-pack-a-day Chesterfield habit buried him and his nicotine-stained fingers in 1977. Mom followed nineteen years later with a worn-out heart. He was sixty-seven, she was eighty-three.

Stephen was nineteen when he died in the hills of North Korea in a December, 1950 ambush. They say that the temperature that winter reached twenty below. Dean is a corporate lawyer in Manhattan. We weren't very close when we were growing up, and we still aren't. My sisters, Dorothy and Melissa, teach school in Jamestown, live on the same block, and see each other almost daily. Dorothy married an electrician, Bernie Madden, twenty-four years ago and they have two kids. Melissa never married, but we think there was a close call back in the early seventies with a hippie from Buffalo she met at a Grateful Dead concert. Every once in a while she hums "Casey Jones" and gets that woulda-coulda-shoulda look in her eyes.

Other than the girls, we are not an especially close family, but we make all the required holiday calls and never forget to send birthday cards. My guess is that we are a fairly typical American family.

As for me, after a three-year stint in the Army and a short-lived marriage— where I saw more combat in the bedroom than I did in the rice paddies of Viet Nam—I used the GI Bill to complete my undergraduate degree in business management at the University of Michigan. As a student in Ann Arbor, I met and fell in love with Laurie Williams. In 1975, with Richard and Karen Carpenter singing "We've Only Just Begun," Laurie and I were married. We have three children—two girls, Audrey and Erica, and our son, Benjamin ("Call me Ben!"). The girls are seventeen and fifteen. Ben is twelve.

Laurie stayed at home until Ben was two and then went back to work as a medical secretary at a local hospital.

Right out of school, I took a job in the personnel department with the Ford Motor Company where I stayed for ten years. In 1986, I made the jump to Erie Shores Ball Bearing. In 1997, I became vice president of Human Resources.

Erie Shores, located in Detroit, is a small, three-shift, industrial company with a steady workforce of about 430. The average age is thirty-seven with an equal mix of men and women. About fifty employees have been here since the company was founded in 1972, and like so many small shops in the area, we rise and fall with the auto industry. There's an old saying around here: "When the nation gets a cold, the auto industry gets pneumonia." Well, when the auto industry gets pneumonia, companies like Erie Ball Bearing die. Currently, Uncle Sam has the sniffles so we're a little on edge.

ONE OF THE BOYS

While friendly, I was never really close to any of the employees until Todd Mersky from shipping shredded his hamstring running to first base. That left our company softball team without a pitcher.

Way back a hundred years ago, I was a pretty good ballplayer, and I still have Walter Mitty dreams of coming to bat in the bottom of the ninth inning, score tied, bases loaded and: "…he swings. There goes a long fly ball to left field, way up there. It's going, going, gone! And McGregor wins the game. The crowd is going wild!"

So, when I heard that they needed someone to pitch, I decided it was time to try for one last triumphant swagger around the bases.

You see, in slow-pitch softball, the pitcher is often the oldest or slowest guy on the team, so I qualified on both accounts—very little running and you don't have to throw the ball too far. Of course, you do have to learn to duck. So, filled with visions of sharp line drives hit up the gap in left-center and the sound of wild applause, I approached the team about stepping in to replace Mersky, and they said, "…Yeah, sure, why not? We can't find anyone else." Not exactly a rousing endorsement, but it got me back on the field. That's when I became One of the Boys.

I enjoy the camaraderie of being part of a team and I enjoy the simple thrill of playing the game. The kid in me likes rolling in the dirt and swinging for the fences while the older guy—reeking of Ben Gay and thankful for ACE Bandages—appreciates the beer after the game and the lies you get to tell about when you were a kid and could really play ball. Over time, the guys have grown to think of me more as their softball teammate and less as "McGregor from HR." They even let me join them for lunch.

LUNCH WITH THE "A" TEAM

Before joining the softball team, I usually skipped lunch or went out with a few of the senior staff. However, to be honest, the other folks on the management team bore me. I was tired of the same old routine. So, when Ted Johnson from sales (a great third baseman) invited me to join him and a few of the other guys at their lunch table, I jumped at the chance. I felt like I was at Jamestown High School all over again, but this time the "A" table wanted me to sit with them! Soon, lunch with these guys became a regular and welcome part of my day. We talked about sports, food, wives and girlfriends, kids, drugs, getting older, and our softball war injuries. You know—guy stuff.

It's because of these lunch talks that I now suspect that, while men and women might be from the same species, there is some pretty compelling evidence that we dropped out of different trees. You be the judge.

YOU'RE INVITED

Now, it's my turn to do the inviting. I invite you to be my guest every Friday for the next fifteen weeks. Listen carefully and you will hear bravado, sensitivity, brilliance, fear, kindness, stupidity, compassion, anger, and sadness. Professor Edwards from the university, a self-professed Mickey Mantle expert, and The Mick, himself, will join us. Professor Edwards will elaborate, clarify, and correct any of the health issues discussed, and Mickey will offer what the broadcast media would call "color commentary" and expert coaching. For those of you who are not familiar with Mickey Mantle, I invite you to go back and re-read the Introduction to this book.

PLAYERS, ROLES, AND PURPOSE

The following is a listing of our players (including me). The descriptions capture start-of-the-season character traits, as well as the typical male concerns we represent. In some cases, the descriptions foreshadow what happens during the season.

Tom McGregor, age fifty-four, Human Resources Department
Primary Role: Narrator

I represent the typical former jock that is now a "weekend warrior." (Actually, my battlefield is the Thursday Night Municipal Softball League.) On the ball field, I have the spirit of a twelve-year-old, but unfortunately, I can't exchange my middle-aged body. As mentioned earlier, I am married for the second time with two teenaged girls and a pre-teen son. The kids are from my second marriage. I have a relatively stable home life and am in good general health.

While I am new to the lunch group, I seem to receive more than my fair share of deference and respect. This is probably due to my title, age, and gray hair, but I like to think it's because of my brilliant play on the diamond and my powerful charisma. All right, most likely it is due to my title, age, and gray hair. In the group, I tend to listen more than talk, although I occasionally bring up new topics and, when asked, I offer my frank and honest opinion.

Concerns

Like a lot of guys my age, I am becoming a bit too cautious and complacent. Where there was once fire, there appears to be only burning embers—actually smoldering ash is more like it, kind of like charcoal four hours after the last burnt cheeseburger has been scraped off the grill. This tepid condition applies to my home life as well as work. Everything is fine, just not very exciting.

The softball playing and after-game time with these guys helps, but I still feel an emptiness I can't seem to fill. Also, truth be told, I'm not in as good a condition as these guys think I am. I'm starting to feel some sharp pain in my knees and I am concerned about pulling a muscle, breaking something, or worse, making a fool out of myself. Two more things: I'm not real pleased with the amount of sunscreen needed for the top of my head, and my stream isn't what it used to be—if you know what I mean. Over the course of the season, I facilitate the following men's health issues:
- Male "Menopause"
- Prostate Cancer
- Sports Injuries

Ted Johnson, age twenty-eight, Sales & Marketing Department
Primary Role: Seducer

Ted has too much charm for his own good. He covers fear with bravado, sexual flirtations, and one-dimensional relationships.

A good salesperson, Ted is able to see things through the eyes of the customer. He is able to find out what they want and what they care about. He asks questions, does not make assumptions, and gives the appearance of being sincerely interested in the concerns of others. Ted likes being his own boss, making his own hours, and meeting new people. He is self-motivated with high energy. With his charm, good looks, and talent, he has the potential to be a strong leader in his community. Of course, it takes more than charm, good looks, and talent to be a real leader.

Concerns

Ted is a little too friendly and manipulative. Also, he is the last to leave the bar after the games and he doesn't always leave alone. At the office, what was once charming and harmless sexual banter is beginning to wear thin. Guys are raising their eyebrows and the women are talking. Ted is twenty-eight, married, and has two small children. Over the course of the season, Ted facilitates the following men's health issues:
- Alcoholism
- Philandering
- Sexual Harassment

Jim Eveshevski, age forty-four, Product Engineering
Primary Roles: Doubting Thomas, Victim, and Beacon of Hope

Jim graduated with honors from Purdue University and immediately went to work for Erie Shores. He is in his mid-forties and is very analytical and objective. On average, Jim shows a healthy skepticism before committing to a position. Pretty much of a Joe Friday kind of a guy ("The facts, ma'am, just the facts"), he is mechanically gifted but not so gifted when it comes to expressing his feelings. You get a sense from Jim that, like an iceberg, you only see a small part of who he really is.

Concerns

A combination of unfulfilled dreams, an inability to express honest emotions, and challenging home circumstances are changing a healthy skeptic into a distrustful cynic. Where Jim used to show at least some minor variation in moods, his affect lately is best described as flat. Also, we have to almost beg Jim to join us for a cold one after a game ("Pepsi, please"). Jim's been married for almost twenty years and has two teenaged daughters and a sick, live-in mother-in-law. His dad committed suicide five years ago, but he's never discussed it. Fact is, I rarely hear him mention his family at all, and when he does his remarks are tinged with the only emotion he ever shows lately—quiet resentment. Over the course of the season, Jim facilitates the following men's health issues:

• Depression
• Suicide
• Parenting

Lou Stevens (Big Lou), age thirty-eight, Shipping and Receiving
Primary Role: Clown and "Ostrich" (Master of Denial)

"The Big Guy" all his life, Lou is friends with the whole world. If the mood gets too tense or too serious, people look to Lou to find a way to lighten things up. He is the proverbial Life of the Party and a pleasure to be around. He has never married, has no children, and lives alone but doesn't appear to be lonely.

Everything Lou does is super-sized including drinking, smoking, and, most of all, eating whenever and whatever possible. Lou's motto: "No steak too thick, no pie too sweet, and no beer too cold!" Also, at 6'2", 280 lbs., with a great eye, his towering home runs are legendary with the Municipal softball crowd. He can hit a ball farther than any man I know. Problem is that he has to. With all that weight, he can barely run out a line drive to the corner in left field. Also, he has been known to light up a Camel as soon as he reaches base and keep one going throughout the game.

Concerns

Lou is a life-long bachelor who thinks that "self-care" means that he has to make his own macaroni and cheese. He hacks all the time and his breathing is getting really labored. Lately, it seems that he has one continuous cold. When you bring up his three-pack-a-day Camel habit, he just laughs and asks, "Got a light?" Other than softball, he never walks when he can ride and never, *ever* climbs stairs if there's an elevator or escalator going his way. After a long walk from the parking lot, he sits down and wheezes and sputters like the last spit from a near empty can of whipped cream. He gave up cooking years ago and knows all the specials at McDonald's. Lois Walters, our company nurse, tells him every other week to cut down on sodium, but he just laughs his husky, smoker's laugh and says, "Pass the salt!" Over the course of the season, Lou facilitates the following men's health issues:
  • Denial
  • Obesity
  • Hypertension
  • Lung Cancer
  • Emphysema
  • Heart Disease
  • Stroke

Troy Phillips, age twenty-two, Information Technology
Primary Role: Combatant, Young Turk

Troy is a computer whiz kid who can't find his socks. He is naïve and the target of many wink-wink-nudge-nudge jokes. He breezed through his undergraduate work at Michigan Tech in less than three years. Would have been faster, according to Troy, but he had to take "moronic" classes like *The History of Western Civilization* and *English 101* ("What a complete waste of time").

Troy lives like a kid at college who no longer has to worry about Mom and Dad sneaking into his room and going through his stuff. A fast car, a Harley Hog, lots of girl friends, a billfold filled with credit cards, an impressive string of weekend binges and the absolute belief that he is invincible—these are the things that mark and measure his life. Troy is James Dean meets Bill Gates.

Troy is brilliant, angry, reckless, and naïve. He is arrogant with a disarming mix of innocence and charm. He has an absolute disregard for caution and lives life on the edge. To add to this disturbing picture, he objectifies women and thinks of them as inferior. He's a hell of a second baseman, but the young man is headed for trouble. Thank God he's single and doesn't have any children.

Concerns

It's fun, at times, to watch Troy's zest for life, but his Rebel-Without-a-Cause lifestyle is wearing thin. He often jumps on his bike without a helmet, thinks that a tan is "cool," has a slew of speeding tickets, and his bursts of temper at the softball games are as well known as Lou's belly laughs. At the slightest provocation, he goes off like a roman candle. Also, while many of us secretly enjoy the portal view of his sexual conquests, I question whether or not it is just his socks that he sometimes forgets to wear. He's a potential biohazard in leather. No problems at work, per se, but I have this growing gut feeling that he is flirting with disaster. Over the course of the season, Troy facilitates the following men's health issues:

- Accidents
- Misogyny
- Fear of Intimacy
- Skin and Testicular Cancer
- Sexually Transmitted Disease
- Financial Difficulties
- Substance Abuse
- Diminished Work Performance

Chris Iverson, age thirty-two, Health Promotion Specialist
Primary Roles: Know-It-All, Agitator, and Facilitator

Chris is an exercise physiologist in charge of our Fitness Center. A former college gymnast, Chris is the resident wellness guru (or "Wellness Nazi," according to some). He is well trained and educated when it comes to exercise physiology and health promotion. However, he often misses the boat when it comes to understanding personal motivation and the dynamics of human behavior.

As the director of the fitness center, Chris coordinates our annual physicals, produces a monthly newsletter called, "Health: It's Up to You!" and offers a variety of programs to lose weight, quit smoking, and manage stress. He also maintains an extensive wellness library. I'm sure if you asked him, he would tell you that he does much more than that—and I'm sure he does. To say Chris is intolerant, rigid, and condescending to the "unwell" masses is like saying that a politician likes to kiss babies and smile for the camera. He means well, but he's arrogant, condescending, and never seems to let up.

The fact that Chris and Troy are on the same team is a perfect example of how softball attracts all kinds—you could not ask for more different personalities. Fact is, Chris barely tolerates any of us. My guess is that he joins us for lunch because he views the group in much the same way that a seventeenth-century missionary looked at a population of "heathens." We represent a challenge. The fact that we play softball gives him hope.

Chris is married to an attorney and they have a three-year-old boy that they adopted at birth.

Concerns

Chris is like the worst reformed smoker who goes around putting out other people's cigarettes with a squirt gun. He actually did that to Big Lou—once. In fact, he is so rigid and intolerant that he turns off many would-be fitness folks. His direct supervisor has spoken to him about this, but he just doesn't seem to get it. It really is a shame because I like Chris. However, his lack of tolerance for slackers may lead to trouble. High scores for book smarts but, as we move into the next fifteen weeks of the season, he gets a failing mark for emotional intelligence. Over the course of the season, Chris facilitates the following men's health issues:

- Hubris
- Workplace Alienation/Isolation
- Over-Training
- Growth

chapter
two

Rough Night...
Alcohol, Steroids, Marijuana, Guy Talk, and Male Bonding

The team comes together this morning, gathering their bruised egos and mopping up after the previous evening's sound thrashing on the softball diamond. We quickly move to a banter-and-bravado discussion of Ted's post-game beer drinking and carousing. Not only does Ted defend his drinking, he rationalizes that a good salesman needs to know how to "booze and schmooze" with his clients. Besides, says Ted, "Beer is good for you." He quotes studies suggesting that alcohol reduces the risk of heart attacks and that beer is a good source of carbohydrates and will therefore help boost energy levels before and after training sessions. Chris, the "Wellness Nazi," jumps all over Ted and trashes all drinking "...other than an occasional glass of Merlot." As for chasing after young girls, Lou weighs in, but Ted pays little attention to Lou's obvious disgust.

The conversation moves to performance-enhancing drugs and their impact on athletes like the East German swimmers, the Canadian sprinter, Ben Johnson, and football star Lyle Alzado who died from brain cancer and blamed his disease on habitual use of steroids.

Predictably, Troy takes a very cavalier attitude, Chris goes ballistic, Lou lives in a world where tobacco and booze are okay but "real" drugs are for losers. Jim is almost too quiet, and I play Devil's Advocate.

At the end of lunch, the guys go back to banter and jokes to offset the serious tone

In the commentary section, Mickey tells the story of how he got hooked on booze and what it did to his life. He also talks about his son Billy's addiction to painkillers, and his son Danny's use of cocaine. Mickey includes a couple of stories that may have, at one time, seemed glamorous and funny. Now, in contrast to how his life turned out, they just seem sad. Professor Edwards gives us the clinical picture.

To say last night's game was one-sided is like Custer saying Little Big Horn was a disappointment. We got our butts kicked, 22–3. If you know much about slow-pitch softball you realize how difficult it is for a team to only score three runs. So, it is with our tails tucked securely between our legs that we gather for lunch.

I break the ice. "Damn, we really stunk up the park last night!"

Nobody bites, they just mumble and look at their food. "Well…" I say, "at least nobody got hurt." At which point Lou laughs and says, "Not unless you count Ted fallin' off his stool at Annie's!"

"Again," says Troy without looking up.

"Christ, Ted," Lou continues, "you musta' guzzled a sixer in less than an hour. How the hell can you drink like that and still make it to work the next morning? And, by the way, who was that redhead you were harassing at the bar? She coulda' been your daughter, for Christ's sake. What the hell's the matter with you?"

Ted says, flashing his famous salesman's smile, "I was just giving the young lady the momentary joy of my company. And, as for her name, I can't remember.

"Now, with regard to my tolerance for Heinekens, chalk it up to prime physical conditioning, my friends, prime physical conditioning. Besides, a brewski now and then is good for your heart. Ain't that right, Doc?"

"Don't call me Doc," says Chris for the gazillionth time. "Actually, a beer now and then is fine. But don't kid yourself about booze and heart disease. There are plenty of other ways to take care of your heart." With an ever so slight smile, Chris glances at Lou. "Like not eating three cheeseburgers and an extra order of fries each day for dinner."

"Screw you, Doc," spits out Lou, along with bits of his triple-decker bologna and cheese sandwich. "You're just jealous 'cause I'm prettier than you."

Lou and Chris trade jabs like this on a regular basis. While there is always a bit of an edge to their exchanges you get the sense that, on some level, they would like to be a little bit like the other. Chris needs to lighten up a bit and Lou knows that he needs to slow down the daily loads of fat, salt, and sugar. Our very own Odd Couple.

"And do you have to spray your food *every* time you talk?"

"Screw you…CHRIS. Oh, so sorry. Wouldy'a please toss back the bologna? I'll need it later, for a snack."

Ignoring their exchange of barbs, Troy speaks, "Yeah, what's up with that, anyhow? I heard that beer is a good source of carbs and vitamins."

"You're better off drinking pop if you want hollow carbs. And with pop it takes longer to screw up your liver and fry your brain," says Chris.

"Too late for Troy," adds Lou.

Again, without moving his head, Troy shoots back, "So, when are you scheduled for that heart and liver transplant, Big Guy?"

The conversation moves off liquor and leads to a discussion of athletes and steroids.

By the way, I'm always amazed at how us guys say so much without saying anything. I recently read that men and women listen differently. According to this study, men listen with only one side of their brains, while women use both. That may explain our tendency to speak in short bursts and in code. Of course, women are having a field day with this report.

"Hey, Doc," says Lou with an emphasis on *Doc* and a wink toward Ted, "could McGwire, Sosa, and Bonds hit all them home runs if they weren't taking steroids?"

Chris shoots back, "You moron, there's no proof that Sosa and Bonds take steroids. And McGwire took andro for a while when he was playing, but he stopped when the press began to squawk. Besides, did you ever see a McGwire home run? He maybe got a few feet deeper with a supplement but, damn, that guy hit the ball 500 feet! No steroid will do that. He was just a natural moose."

Softly, Jim speaks for the first time, "Remember that sprinter from Canada who won the gold medal and later tested positive for steroids? What was his name?"

"Ben Johnson," answers Chris, with authority.

"What ever happened to him?" asks Ted.

"Last I heard, he was giving fitness training to Moammar Gadhafi's son," says Chris.

"So, who's he play for, this Gadhafi guy?" asks Lou.

Chris can only shake his head. The others smile.

"How about Lyle Alzado?" asks Chris.

"Football, Oakland, tough guy," says Lou. "What about him?"

"Alzado was diagnosed with brain cancer in the early 1990s and became convinced that his twenty-year use of steroids and growth hormones had caused his illness," says Chris. He looks at Lou and waves his fork around, "Now, that's stupid. He even admitted it was dumb before he died."

Lou smiles as he sees an opening, "All right, okay, so, it's two o'clock in the morning and a husband and his wife are asleep when suddenly the phone rings. The husband picks up the phone and says 'Hello?...How the hell do I know? What am I, the weather man?' He promptly slams the phone down. His wife rolls over and asks, 'Who was that?' The husband replies, 'I don't know, it was some guy who wanted to know if the coast was clear.' Now, that's stupid!...Pass the salt." Lou laughs at his own joke.

I'll ask Mickey and Dr. Edwards to comment on this later, but the whole male bonding scene is really pretty fascinating to watch. Why is it that so many of us men show affection with insults, puff out our chests when threatened and, inevitably, bring the conversation around to cars, electronic gadgets, booze, sports, the stock market, or women?

"Why don't you just inject that poison?" says Chris.

"Hey, at least I don't smoke no dope or do drugs, like half of the degenerates around here! Oh, sorry, Troy, no offense."

Wrapped in a sardonic chuckle, Troy shoots Lou the finger.

"Wait a minute, let me get this straight," says Chris. "You don't think that those Camels you smoke or the beer you drink are drugs? Is that what you're saying?"

"Damn straight, that's what I'm saying. They're both legal."

"I swear, Lou, you drive me nuts. Nicotine is more addictive than heroin, and alcohol is not only addictive, it's an addiction that can be inherited. Hell, eating your five cheeseburgers a day is more harmful than Troy smoking an occasional joint!"

"Yeah, well, up yours, Lycra Boy. And, Troy, there, smokes more dope than I smoke Camels. Christ, look at his eyes. He probably just toked-up before lunch and was planning on another for dessert!"

Everyone looks at Troy who just laughs even harder than Lou. He laughs just a little bit too hard and definitely too long.

Now, remember while we have been eating lunch and shooting the bull, Mickey and the Professor have been listening in and taking notes—well, at least the Professor has been taking notes. After each lunch, I will sit with these two guys and discuss what was said. Also, in case you hadn't guessed, I cleaned up the language a bit. My teammates, particularly Lou, can get pretty raunchy. Actually, to be honest, that's part of his charm.

What Would Mickey Say?
About Alcohol, Male Bonding, and Steroids

Tom: Listening to these guys, Mick, what comes to mind?

Mickey: Well, to tell the truth, I can relate to Lou, he seems like a good ol' boy that knows how to have a good time—same with Ted. Problem is that what seems like a good idea at the moment can come back and bite you in the butt. Right now, Ted is having fun flirting with the girls and chugging beer, but, hey, I've been there; he's playing with matches, and sooner or later that guy's going to get burned. And, that probably goes for Lou, too. I'm not sure about Troy, but it sounds like he might be running a bit too free and wild. As for Chris, he seems like a Bobby Richardson[1] kind of a guy—pretty straight-laced and goes by the book. Only difference is that Bobby was always nice and never tried to put anyone down. Chris seems kind of mean and ornery.

Tom: You were known to have closed a few bars in your day. How did a kid from Commerce, Oklahoma become such a party guy?

Mickey: When I came up with the Yankees in 1951, I was only nineteen years old. I arrived in New York with a cardboard suitcase and one sport coat. I never knew what to say, and girls made me blush. Other than a beer now and then, I hardly drank at all. My dad, Mutt Mantle, didn't drink much either. He would buy a half-pint and sip on it for days. Shoot, when I was a kid, he woulda' whipped my fanny if he caught me taking a drink.

Then when he died the next spring of Hodgkin's disease, I was devastated. Hell, he was only thirty-nine years old! I think I started to drink heavily to deal with the pain of losing him.

Tom: And the partying?

Mickey: As for partying and having fun, it didn't take long before Billy[2] and Whitey[3] helped me get over some of my shyness. When we went to the bars there was sort of a contest to see who could flirt with the most girls and who could hold the most liquor. It was all about male bonding stuff; you know—we were buddies. It was what you were supposed to do.

Honest to God, we were like rock stars. The temptations were everywhere. Every guy wanted to buy you a drink and plenty of gals wanted to, well, you know....

That was part of being a man. Drink good booze, eat a thick steak, make time with the girls, stay out late, and then go play baseball the next day. Shoot, it was the American Dream for any guy! And, as long as we won, nobody gave us a hard time. In fact Casey[4] used to say that, yeah, some of his stars drank whiskey, but he found that the ones who drank milkshakes didn't win many ballgames.

Part of the problem was I didn't get hung over. I always felt great the next day—ready to go play ball. Like Ted, there, I had a tremendous tolerance for alcohol.

Tom: How did it make you feel, the alcohol?

Mickey: Without the booze, I was still a shy kid from Oklahoma who just wanted to play baseball. It was all I lived for, to play baseball, but with a couple of drinks, hell, I was Mickey Mantle! People laughed at my jokes, guys picked up my bar tab, and the ladies wanted to dance and fool around. It wasn't until later that it really messed with my mind and screwed up my life.

Tom: When did it catch up with you?

Mickey: That's one of the problems with alcohol. At least for me, there was no one moment when I felt I lost control; it just kind of snuck up and grabbed me. To show how much I was in control, I would periodically call a "time out" and go for a couple of weeks without a drink. That way, I knew I wasn't an alcoholic—I could stop anytime I wanted to.

Man, what a fool I was. I wish I could go back and find that twenty-year-old Mickey Charles Mantle and talk some sense into him.

Tom: What would you say?

Mickey: Well, I'm not so good with words, but if I could be like those ghosts in the Scrooge story, there are a few scenes I would show him.

Tom: What scenes?

Mickey: There are more horrible scenes than I care to remember, but the ones that hurt the most are the ones with Merlyn[5] and the boys. I'd like the young Mickey Mantle to see the time I thought Merlyn locked me out of the house when I went out drinking with my buddies. As it turned out she didn't, but I was so drunk and mad when she showed up at the house, I yelled at her and roughed her up in front of everyone. Merlyn was pregnant and gave birth to our son, David, just two days later.

Then there was the time Merlyn and me went out with Yogi and Carmen[6] for a nice dinner. I got real drunk and Merlyn didn't want me to drive and Yogi warned her not to ride with me. With Merlyn in the car, I drove anyway and hit a telephone pole. Both of us were pretty shook up but we could have died.

Another time, we were out with Clete Boyer[7] and his wife. I pulled the chair back just as Merlyn was about to sit down—you know, a stupid kid prank. Well, Merlyn fell to the ground and got pretty mad…and hurt. In fact, she left the restaurant, and when I chased her outside, she tried to run me down with our new Oldsmobile. By the time I finally got home, I passed out on the lawn and stayed there for the night.

Boy, this is hard. But, I guess I would want the twenty-year-old Mickey Charles Mantle to see and hear me make a fool of myself in restaurants, being rude to fans, slurring my words, and sometimes crying myself to sleep because I was so scared I was going to die and, at the same time, wishing I would.

Tom: Mick, did you ever think about what it was doing to your health?

Mickey: Hell no, not when I was a kid like Troy or even when I was Lou's age. Truth is, I never thought I would live long enough to have it catch up to me. Like I said, my dad died at thirty-nine and my grandfather died at forty-one. I also had two uncles who never made it out of their thirties. All of them died from Hodgkin's disease.

I figured, what the hell, I might as well party. Of course, if I knew I was going to live as long as I did, I would have taken better care of myself.[8]

But, like I said, it wasn't just me I was hurting. I would get mean and ornery, even to the kids. That's one of the things I really felt bad about—my kids, my boys. I loved my boys, but between the demands of baseball, my drinking, and my fooling around, I didn't give them the time I should have. I never planned it that way; it just happened. Don't get me wrong, I'm not blaming anyone or anything but me. I'm the one who screwed up. The boys never blamed me and neither did Merlyn or anyone else. They didn't have to.

Tom: What made you decide to stop drinking?

Mickey: A bunch of things, I guess. The older I got, the more alcohol I would drink and the worse I would feel. Some days I would start out with what Billy and I called our "Breakfast of Champions"—a big glass filled with brandy, Kahlua, and cream. I really missed Billy after he died, so sometimes I would have an extra one for him.[9]

Anyway, after a couple of those, it was all over. I would drink the rest of the day until I couldn't drink any more. I'd usually finish with vodka martinis in some restaurant where I would order food but never eat, just drink. It helped me overcome my shyness and put me at ease. Lots of times, I couldn't remember where I had been or what I did. Later, when people told me, I would feel really bad. That would start me thinking that I had a problem and probably should do something about it.

I also started forgetting things and feeling kind of paranoid and depressed. I even moved in with my son, Danny, so I would feel safe.

I think it was when Danny checked into Betty Ford that I really started seriously thinking about quitting. You see, I felt like I was the reason Danny had to go. For years, I would grab Danny, Mickey, Jr., and David and say, "Hey guys, let's go get something to eat." But that really meant let's go drink. I never played catch with my kids; instead when they were old enough I made them my drinking buddies. It reminded me of the old days with Whitey and Billy. I used my boys to keep me company while I drank and I let them watch me sink lower and lower. I pulled them down right along with me too. Yeah, it was probably talking with Danny after his treatment that convinced me to try Betty Ford.[10]

Tom: So that was that? No more drinking?

Mickey: Except for the regrets and the scars, yes. After Betty Ford, no more drinking, just a whole hell of a lot of painful memories and lots of regrets. That's what I would tell the young me. Don't think you can change everything you did and make it all better. You can't. So think—first.

Ah, hell, who would believe a person could be handed his dream on a silver platter and manage to screw it up so much? If someone did show me all this when I was a kid, I probably wouldn't have believed him—even if it were me doing the showing and telling.

Tom: How about steroids, Mick? Did you see any doping in your day?

Mickey: I saw a lot of dopes, if that's what you mean. I was one of them. We drank enough to sink a battleship, smoked cigarettes, and ate tons of fat, but nobody was using steroids. Today's steroid junkies are the real dopes. They don't care that the stuff can make you crazy and even kill you. Yeah, I know you can say the same for booze and tobacco, but we didn't know all the harm we were doing, and, besides, I don't think being drunk or hung over helped me hit any home runs or steal many bases.

Well, actually, there was this time back in 1963 in Baltimore when Whitey and I did some heavy drinking the night before a game. Whitey had just pitched the day before and I thought I was on the disabled list so I figured, no problem, let 'er pour. By the time I got to the park the next day, the only thing that was worse than the way I looked was the way I felt, so I settled in for a nice recovery nap on the bench. Along about the seventh inning, Ralph[11] taps me on the shoulder and asks me if I can hit. Hell, I tell him, I'm not even on the active list.

Ralph says, "You are now, so get up there."

My old Yankee drinking buddy, Hank Bauer[12], was coaching the Orioles and he knew what condition I was in. My guess is that he told the pitcher to just throw bullets and get me out of there. As I walked to the plate, I heard Whitey laugh and tell me to swing at the first fastball. And, that's what I did. I connected, and it flew over the center-field fence. As I passed Brooks Robinson[13] at third base all he could do was shake his head in disbelief and probably a bit of disgust.

Maybe the booze helped me that day because I felt sick and I just wanted to get back to the bench as quickly as possible, but I wouldn't exactly call it a performance-enhancing drug.

Tom: How about marijuana?

Mickey: Yeah, some guys were smoking it, but it wasn't widespread. As far as I was concerned, drugs were for losers and skid row bums. I never touched the stuff. I was a lot like Lou: I had this righteous attitude that said booze was okay because it was legal but anything else was strictly wrong. Hey, by the way, Lou, that's crazy thinking.

Also—about drugs—remember, I played in the 1950s and 1960s. Baseball wasn't any different than the rest of the country at that time. Drugs like marijuana and cocaine were for the most part underground and not so readily available. Of course, drugs hit the baseball world just like the rest of the country beginning in the 1970s and it wasn't long before you could get drugs in any schoolyard or, for Hollywood types and other rich guys, go to a party and have your host serve you your drug of choice.

But it wasn't steroids and marijuana that Whitey, Billy, and I wanted. We wanted liquor and pretty girls. Like I said, we were no different than any other guys back then—except maybe for the fact that we could get plenty of whatever we wanted, or at least, more than the guys in the bleacher seats.

Tom: Anything else you want to say about steroids, marijuana, or any other drugs?

Mickey: Yeah, well, this is very hard to talk about; I want everyone to remember a beautiful young boy named Billy. When this boy was a cancer patient he was so hooked on drugs he would hide prescription pills, grind the pills to powder, mix them in water and inject them into the catheter placed in his chest for the chemo. Billy was my son. Billy was diagnosed with Hodgkin's disease when he was just nineteen. On top of the cancer, he struggled for years with depression, alcohol, and drug abuse, including crack cocaine. He was in and out of treatment centers four times in four years. He was just thirty-six when his heart gave out and he died. At the time, he was under arrest for driving while intoxicated.

So, yes, if it means anything to anyone, I just want to say to the guys like Troy who seem to think that it's cool to walk through life with a marijuana buzz or Ted who thinks nothing of downing a six-pack while scouting young girls, be careful. That's all—just be careful and think about what you're doing. I played that game and lost—worse than that, I hurt other people and pissed away hours, days, weeks, and years of precious moments that could have been spent with my family. I did it. No one forced me. It was no one's fault but mine. A lot of people want to take the blame for how I turned out, make excuses for me. But, truth is, none of us can duck away from the man in the mirror.

Tom, now that I think of it, I guess I have one more scene for that young Mickey Charles Mantle. I want him to peek into the future, hear his voice, and see Merlyn's face when he calls her on the phone and says, "Merlyn...it's about Billy...he's dead." Yeah, I guess I'd want the young me to see that too. Maybe, just maybe, if Billy had a father who was there for him, that call would never have happened.

Tom: I know it's hard to talk about this stuff, Mick, and I appreciate you sharing your story with the readers. So, you heard our lunch gang go at each other pretty hard, but underneath the insults there seems to be some real affection. You had great friendships with teammates and your boys. What was that like?

Mickey: Yeah, guys are funny like that. The more they like each other, the more they trash each other. It's just the way guys are, I guess. I was always calling Billy and Whitey names and playing practical jokes on them, but truth be told, I loved those guys and they knew it. Of course, I never told them that. They'da really razzed me if I did. Well, maybe not. But they would'a felt pretty weird about it. One of things I regret most is the fact that I never even told my dad that I loved him. Never. I guess maybe I was afraid he would think I was weak or a sissy or something like that. Man, I'm sorry I never told him.

The Professor Speaks[14]
About Alcohol, Male Bonding, and Steroids

Tom: Okay, Professor, we heard a lot of noise from the table. What do we believe, what do we toss, and what's missing?

Professor Edwards: I took a lot of notes so let's get right to it. I will take the items one at a time.

ALCOHOL

The good news: alcohol in moderation has health benefits. For example, both regular and light beers offer a significant amount of vitamin B-12, important for vegans (people who eat only plant foods). Red wine is also a good source of dietary iron, a mineral that helps prevent anemia among athletes. Red wine also contains health-protective phenolic compounds that may reduce the risk of heart disease. Wine drinking may partially explain why French people who have been eating a diet rich in saturated fat (the worst kind of fat) have enjoyed better heart-health than might be expected. Wine is certainly not the only reason why France has less death from heart disease, but it is one factor that merits recognition.

Tom: So, what's the bad news?

Professor Edwards: The bad news? Alcohol is the most abused drug in the United States. Prolonged consumption can lead to cellular changes in the liver, heart, brain, and muscle and can result in cirrhosis, pancreatitis, irregular heartbeats, stroke, and malnutrition. Moderate drinkers have a higher risk of oral cancer, and both men and women who drink may have a higher risk of breast cancer. Because alcohol is a highly addictive substance, it has a high potential for abuse and is associated with adverse effects on health and safety.

As for alcohol and athletics, alcohol is a depressant and offers no edge for athletes—apart from killing pain. You can't be sharp, quick, and drunk. Late night partying that contributes to getting too little sleep before the next morning's event creates another problem. Before the game, whatever the game may be, you may want alcohol to calm anxiety, but alcohol has a negative effect on reaction time, hand-eye coordination, accuracy, balance, and overall coordination. It does not improve strength, power, speed, or endurance.

Chris is right. Alcohol is a poor source of carbohydrates. You may get loaded with beer, but your muscles won't get carbo-loaded. A twelve-ounce can of beer has only fourteen grams of carbs, as compared to forty grams in a can of soft drink.

Alcohol is absorbed directly from the stomach into the bloodstream, appearing within five minutes after consumption. Post-exercise, alcohol on an empty stomach can quickly contribute to a drunken stupor. Your liver breaks down alcohol at a fixed rate—less than four ounces of wine or a can of beer per hour. Exercise does not hasten that process.

Also, alcohol has a dehydrating effect—bad for athletes—which also leads to bad hangovers. Dehydration is a major problem for many athletes. Water loss of 4 to 5 percent of body weight can result in a 20–30 percent drop in work capacity. At the very least, have one glass of water for every beer. If you are determined to drink—drink moderately. The definition of moderate drinking is two drinks per day for men and one for women.

For you party guys, keep in mind that hot tubs and alcohol are a bad combination. The hotter your body is, the drunker you may get. Alcohol impairs your ability to control your body temperature, plus the high temperature heightens the body's response to alcohol. Cold temperatures are also a problem. Skiing and alcohol is a dangerous duo.

Lou needs to keep in mind that the calories in alcohol are fattening. People who drink moderately tend to consume alcohol calories on top of their regular caloric intake. These excess calories promote body fat accumulation. This helps to explain Lou's beer belly. Also, it's harder to feel full when alcohol becomes a part of the diet because alcohol stimulates the appetite. If you are trying to maintain a lean machine, you're better off abstaining than imbibing.

Keep in mind that as in Mickey's case alcoholism is hereditary. Chris was right about this as well. Also, in the general population drinking problems occur in about 16–24 percent of men and 5 percent of women. This varies with age. People under forty-five years have higher rates of alcohol problems that do older folks. Be conscious of your ability to keep alcohol consumption within socially and medically acceptable bounds. Don't start drinking if you can't easily stop. If you have a parent or grandparent who is—or was—an alcoholic, be extra cautious.

Because of the detrimental effects of alcohol on performance, one might think that serious athletes would be less likely to drink alcohol, but this is not the case. Research shows that college athletes generally out-drink non-athletes. Alcohol-control education programs don't seem to make a difference, as athletes were shown to drink more even though they were quicker to notice messages against drinking.

Some of the research findings suggest that the team atmosphere may help to promote heavy drinking behaviors. Research shows that athletes are more likely than non-athletes to have social conditions that raise the likelihood of binge drinking. And athletes are more likely to say that they and their friends are binge drinkers.

MALE BONDING

Tom: Maybe it's part of the binge drinking, but men also seem to loosen up and talk to each other more after they've had a few. Of course, most of the talk is laced with insults and ribbing. Why is that?

Professor Edwards: It's not just under the influence of alcohol that men behave that way. Look, in about forty-five minutes, we listened to guys who obviously like each other enough to meet for lunch every day, play on the same team, and hang out at the bars together. In that time, we heard the following: "Screw you," "Up yours, Lycra Boy," "You're just jealous 'cause I'm prettier than you," "When's that liver transplant, Big Guy?" "You Moron," "Why don't you just inject that poison?" and "Lou, you drive me nuts." We also had comments about spitting bologna, side glances that spoke volumes, and one "says-it-all" gesture of affection from Troy to Lou.

All group bonding, in any environment, tends to involve a private language of in-jokes, nicknames, catch phrases, and customary gestures. These are all attempts to pursue intimacy. Ironically, with a curl of the lip, a twist of the head, a change in inflection, an aggressive move, and a past filled with bad memories, these gestures (literal and metaphoric) become the stuff that starts serious arguments, leads to fist fights, and starts or continues wars between nations.

Friends can hurl insults, strangers and enemies cannot. Of course, there are cultural and generational differences, but the basic process and intent is the same. For our purposes here at Erie, we will stick to the average U.S. male.

Certainly, there are exceptions. Men can be sensitive, introspective, kind, considerate, honest, straightforward, civilized, and open with their feelings. It's just that, according to my wife and several of my female friends, those brothers are limited in number, stay hidden from public view, and—all too often—turn into Lou once you bring one home.

Women hug, kiss on the cheek, and compliment. Of course, the same exceptions listed above also apply to women. Men, however, shake hands, throw some trash, and wait for the return barbs. The preferred venue is a bar but a sporting event will also work—preferably one where you can also toss down a beer or two while talking about how bad the team is and how next year will be different.

Tom: Not all guys hang out at bars or are sports nuts, though.

Professor Edwards: No bar or athletic event? Okay. The lunchroom, water cooler, shipping dock, or local fast-food eatery will work just fine. For some guys, the talk moves to cars, kids, palm-pilots, big-screen TVs, computers, politics (the fun stuff like corruption and scandals), the stock market, and Suzie from Accounting and her fine-looking derrière. This last one is discussed in much the same way as it was back in junior high school with a wink, nudge, and a muffled chuckle. But, when it comes to discussing issues that expose vulnerabilities (without the benefit of a long history of friendship, a shared crisis like divorce, disease, or significant loss, or a social-lubricant like booze or marijuana), the intimacy-constipated male prefers to cover up with the same mask of denial and bravado that he inherited from his father and his father before him.

What we end up with is the kind of bantering and arguing we see from our lunch bunch—a subtly tempered code that allows males to show interest in one another, to express emotion, to be demonstrative, to reveal their personal beliefs, attitudes and aspirations, and to discover those of their companions. In other words, to become more intimate without acknowledging that this is their objective.

Take for example when Lou said to Ted, "Who was that redhead you were harassing at the bar? She could'a been your daughter, for Christ's sake. What the hell's the matter with you?"

In the mist of the light-hearted jousting, Lou makes his point that he disapproves of Ted's womanizing. He does so with the words and phrases, "harassing," "could'a been your daughter," and "What the hell's the matter with you?" And, if you remember his body language, there was no doubt that he disapproved; however, he stopped just short of a serious confrontation. He did this by tagging the criticism at the end of a smile following a veiled compliment about Ted's ability to handle his liquor. Then, he looked at Ted when he asked about the identity of the redhead, but then looked at the other guys when he said, "She could'a been your daughter, for Christ's sake." Finally, and clearly, he looked right at Ted when he asked, rhetorically, "What the hell's the matter with you?" Everyone at the table knows *exactly* what he means, but that's as far as he will take it. The male code allows only so much personal comment on serious personal matters. Of course, my guess is that last night was not Ted's first flirtation.

Ted's reaction to Lou is classic. He deflects the innuendo about the girl and shows a touch of misogyny—that he really doesn't like women—when he says, "…as for her name, I truly can't remember." He puffs out his chest with the comment about his tolerance for alcohol, quickly changes the subject, and shifts the spotlight off him and onto Chris, making it clear to all that the discussion of his private life is now closed.

Tom, you mentioned that study about how men and women listen differently. That study was presented in a paper in November 2000 at the Eighty-Sixth Scientific Assembly and Annual Meeting of the Radiological Society of North America (RSNA).

The study featured twenty men and twenty women whose brains were scanned while listening to portions of *The Partner*, a John Grisham novel. A majority of the men showed exclusive activity on the left side of the brain, in the temporal lobe, which is classically associated with listening and speech. The majority of women showed activity in the temporal lobe on both sides of the brain, although predominantly on the left. The right side of the brain traditionally is associated with performing music and understanding spatial relationships, rather than listening. More and more often it seems that normal for men may be different than normal for women.

The finding may help with research regarding how men and women recover from stroke and brain tumors. It may also help guide brain surgeons in avoiding certain areas of the brain, depending on whether they're operating on men or women. It may also help explain why, when men and women speak in their respective codes, the other sex just doesn't seem to "get it."

FEMALE BONDING

Professor Edwards: It might help men to know that women also have bonding rituals. While not the focus of this discussion, there is one female-bonding practice that bears some surface resemblance to the male argument rituals. Participants in the complimenting ritual do challenge and contradict each other's statements, but almost opposite from the way us men do it. There is no competitiveness and no one-upmanship—in fact, the exchange could be described as an exercise in one-downmanship.

The subject of this ritual conversation is immaterial. You will recognize the complimenting ritual by its structure, which is always the same. It starts with one participant paying another participant a compliment. Etiquette requires the recipient of the compliment to respond with a self-deprecating denial and then another compliment in return. This must immediately be countered with a self-critical denial and a further compliment, which is then denied by the recipient, who pays another compliment in return...and so on.

Again, this is not always the case; however, it is enough so that most women will agree and recognize the dance.

For men who may nod their heads and say that they know exactly what I mean, they're wrong. Women tend to restrain their complimenting ritual when men are around. We never get the full version. To do so, we need to accompany a group of women to the ladies' room...not recommended.

GUY TALK

When Chris says to Lou when talking about heart disease:
"Yeah, like not eating three cheeseburgers and an extra order of fries each day for dinner."
What he really wants to say is:
"I care about you, you big lug. Keep eating like you do and you're dead."

When Lou says to Chris:
"Screw you, Doc. You're just jealous 'cause I'm prettier than you."
What he really wants to say is:
"Thanks for caring."

When Lou says to the table after Chris makes reference to liquor wasting your liver and heavy drugs frying your brain:
"Too late for Troy."
What he really wants to say is:
"Troy, buddy, you're acting goofier and goofier every day and I'm worried about your use of drugs."

When Troy says to Lou:
"So, when are you scheduled for that heart and liver transplant, Big Guy?"
What he really wants to say is:
"I may smoke weed, but you abuse alcohol and you're obese, so don't throw stones in that glass house of yours."

And then, there are times when guys say exactly what they want to say...

When Chris says to Lou:
"You moron, there's no evidence that Sosa and Bonds take steroids."
What he really wants to say is:
"You moron, there's no evidence that Sosa and Bonds take steroids."

When Lou says to Chris:
"Up Yours, Lycra Boy."
What he really wants to say is:
"Up Yours, Lycra Boy."

Tom: And what about tobacco?
Professor Edwards: I'll get to that another day, but for now, let's look at steroids.

STEROIDS

In general terms, steroids are a large group of naturally occurring and synthetic fat-soluble chemicals, with a great diversity of physiological activity. Included among the steroids are certain alcohols (sterols), bile acids, many important hormones, some natural drugs, and even the poisons found in the skin of some toads.

The misconception is that steroids are bad. Of course, they are not "bad." They are a natural component of both plant and animal life and provide numerous medical benefits. For example, most oral contraceptives are synthetic steroids consisting of female sex hormones that inhibit ovulation. Perhaps the most widely used steroids in medicine are cortisone and various synthetic derivatives of this substance. Such steroids are prescription drugs used for a variety of skin ailments, rheumatoid arthritis, asthma and allergies, and various eye diseases, and in cases of adrenal insufficiency, or the malfunctioning of the adrenal cortex.

Lou asked Chris about Mark McGwire and his use of androstenedione, or andro as it's called in the gym. If you want to know the technical description, here it is: androstenedione is a major precursor of both estrogen (a female estrogenic hormone) and the male hormone, testosterone. Your body makes androstenedione from some progesterone and some DHEA. It's one of sixteen human-manufactured hormones in the steroid family tree, all stemming from cholesterol, a vital substance for human functioning. Without cholesterol, there is neither estrogen nor testosterone.

The androgens are the male sex hormones. The principal androgen, testosterone, is produced primarily by the testes and in lesser amounts by the adrenal cortex and, in women, by the ovaries. Androgens are primarily responsible for the development and maintenance of reproductive function and stimulation of the secondary sex characteristics in the male. Androgens also have an anabolic (synthesizing and constructive, rather than degradative) function in stimulating the production of skeletal muscles and bone as well as red blood cells. To enhance the anabolic activity of androgens without increasing their masculinizing ability, anabolic steroids were developed. Though originally intended to combat diseases marked by wasting, individuals desiring to increase their muscle mass, such as athletes seeking to gain a competitive advantage, have abused these synthetic hormones. Overdosing has been linked to serious side effects, including infertility, personality disorders, baldness, severe acne, and coronary heart disease. However, in spite of numerous health warnings and strict bans on the use of anabolic steroids in most professional and amateur sports, we still see widespread use.

Tom: Yeah, but the belief is always that it will happen to the other guy, not me. Do you think if an athlete really thought they were in danger that they would still use steroids?

Professor Edwards: Tom, here is a scenario from a 1995 poll of 198 sprinters, swimmers, power lifters, and other assorted athletes, most of them U.S. Olympians or aspiring Olympians: You are offered a banned performance-enhancing substance, with two guarantees: 1) You will not be caught. 2) You will win. Would you take the substance?

One hundred and ninety-five athletes said yes; three said no.

Here's another scenario offered to the same group: You are offered a banned performance-enhancing substance that comes with two guarantees: 1) You will not be caught. 2) You will win every competition you enter for the next five years, and then you will die from the side effects of the substance. Would you take it?

More than half the athletes said yes.[15]

Jim asked about Ben Johnson, the Canadian sprinter who won the 100-meter dash in the 1988 Olympic Games in Seoul and later was stripped of his medal when he tested positive for banned steroids. Well, if you ask Ben Johnson he will tell you that there is no difference in what Mark McGwire was doing with andro and what he was doing in Seoul. Both were trying to be the best at what they do. The difference, or course, is that, at the time, McGwire was not breaking a rule and Johnson was. However, both were putting their health at risk.

MARIJUANA

Tom: With all this talk of alcohol and drugs, where does marijuana fit in?

Professor Edwards: As discussed by the guys at the lunch table, marijuana refers to the dried flowers and leaves of the Indian hemp plant smoked or eaten as a drug. When taken it tends to heighten perception and relax the body. Actually, I have some concern about Troy and marijuana. When you look closely, he has classic signs of a chronic user—bloodshot eyes, dilated pupils, lack of coordination and energy. Other symptoms include decreased concentration, memory problems, and rapid heart rate.

When you look at Dr. Jack Henningfield's chart of popular drugs, marijuana falls considerably lower on the addiction scale when compared to the other drugs. In fact, it ranks sixth out of six. This in no way suggests that marijuana is safe. In fact, as an unregulated substance there is the potential for great harm. Street dealers, looking to sell the "best" product, are known to peddle marijuana that is laced with LSD, cocaine, heroine, and 1-(1-phencyclohexyl) piperidine— pcp, aka "angel dust" or "zoot." Serious consequences can result, including front temporal lobe seizures leading to a life-long seizure disorder. Users need to beware and know their source. Better yet, leave it alone.

Assuming that the marijuana is pure and not tainted, there are still concerns and cautions. Judgment is impaired in much the same fashion as alcohol and, while not strongly addictive in the physical sense, it can become psychologically habit forming and disruptive. Lethargy, forgetfulness, and reduced sex drive are common side effects associated with habitual use. And, for the record, it's illegal.

Tom: That brings us to lunch, itself. What do think of our diet?

Professor Edwards: I tell you what, let's pick that up another time. I have to get back to the university. Besides, my sense is that Lou will give us ample time to discuss nutrition.

chapter
three

"No Pain, No Gain" and Other Stupid Notions
Muscles, Feet, Joints, Exercise, Stretching, and Common Sense

*W*e start out with Troy making an "old man" comment as he watches me
walk to the table. With the end of an unraveling ACE bandage sticking out my pant
leg, I do my best to avoid limping, but it's no use—what the stiff walk doesn't say,
the grimace on my face does. I confess to the pulled muscle (from two games ago),
but hold back admitting to my other aches and pains. The group is then off on a
discussion of injuries. Mickey Mantle, Nolan Ryan, Cal Ripken, and Joe Namath
are presented in the context of performance, conditioning, and disability.

Troy, twenty years old and a natural "flat-belly," is consistent with his lack of
interest in something as mainstream as stretching and regular exercise. Ted, always
concerned about looking good, concentrates only on what the eyes can see—lots
of sit-ups for that six-pack stomach and arm curls so he can flex for the ladies.
Chris has some good advice about drinking fluids and the importance of stretching.
However, Chris is still far from the perfect role model. For example, when he misses
his daily six-mile run, his mood becomes foul and he fixates on how miserable he
feels. Other revelations suggest the possibility that Chris may be suffering from
"body fixation." No narcissistic worries about Lou, however. He jokes that he gets
plenty of exercise lifting a beer can and walking to the store for smokes.

Professor Edwards picks up on Chris' unhealthy attention to body image and
the dangers of over-training. In Chris' favor, he agrees with the self-proclaimed

fitness guru's scientific rationale for drinking lots of water and keeping muscles and joints limber. Also, among other things, the good professor discusses the dangers associated with "playing hurt," neglecting some muscle groups while favoring others, and the phenomenon of exercise depression. Mickey talks about the pressure professional athletes are under to perform and what it feels like to play day after day with pain. One of his least favorite topics, Mickey talks about how good he might have been had he taken better care of himself.

"Hey, Pops, I'm halfway tempted to set off a false alarm just to watch you run!"

Troy's grin and wise-guy chuckle does nothing to brighten my day. Ever since the massacre on Diamond 3, I have been hobbling around like an old man—a very, very, sore old man. The muscle-pull in my hamstring happened when I tried to stretch a God-given-gift of a double into a triple. A triple! Hell, twenty, no, *thirty* years ago, I didn't have the speed to leg out a triple. What made me think I could do it on the shady side of fifty? Getting thrown out by ten steps was bad enough but to add injury to insult, I now have to deal with a pulled muscle…and the harassment.

Limping to the lunch table, I throw one of those affectionate "screw-you" smiles at Troy.

"Troy!" shouts Lou so everyone can hear, "I bet you a bag of chips that I can eat my hamburger before ol' Tommy-Boy makes it to the table."

"Yeah, Lou," says Troy, "and, let's see, that would mean only two more burgers, an order of fries, a piece of apple pie, and a bag of carrot sticks left on your tray. By the way, what's up with the carrot sticks?"

"I've decided to eat healthy meals," grins Lou sporting a catsup beauty mark just left of his upper lip.

And, so begins Friday's lunch.

"How bad is your leg?" asks Chris.

Not wanting to look like a wimp, I tell him that it's just fine and fall into my lunch chair while squeezing back the tears.

"So, what are you doing for it?"

"You know," I say, "the regular stuff. At first, lots of ice and a couple of Advil. I have it wrapped in a wide ACE bandage."

"We noticed," says Ted with a grin.

"Try to keep off it as much as possible over the next few days," says Chris, "and if the swelling is down, try a heating pad or hot baths along with the Advil.

Also, try very gentle stretching in a day or so to keep from stiffening up. If you'd stretch like you're supposed to, this probably wouldn't have happened.

"One more thing," adds Chris, "drink plenty of water, every day. It will help the new tissue. Also, given your age, Tom, it might be a good idea to skip the next game and give your leg lots of time to heal."

"Hey, Doc," spits Lou, "given *your* age, you might want to show a bit more respect for the old man. He doesn't have very many years to go before—well, you know…"

"Thanks, Lou," I smile.

"Damn," says Troy ogling me and Jim, "I hope I never get as old as you guys. You're just like my ol' man. He's going bald, can't see for crap, got more aches and pains than body parts, can't stay up past ten o'clock without nodding off, and when he does go to sleep he gets up every hour to pee! Shoot me, if I ever get like that!"

"How old is your dad?" I ask.

"Fifty-seven. Mom's fifty-five."

"Ah, yes," I say, "ancient, both of them."

Without looking up from his Brussels sprouts, Chris comments, "It's lifestyle, plain and simple. Take care of your body and it will take care of you. Plain and simple."

"Yeah," says Troy with a smirk, "plain and simple, Chris. Just like you."

We all laugh. Surprisingly, that includes Chris. "Hey, laugh all you want, but it's true. With regular exercise, stretching, and proper diet, there's no reason why you can't be playing softball, or golfing, or skiing when you're in your seventies or even older. Even you, Jim."

Always quiet, but more so the last month or so, Jim doesn't even bother to look up. "Hell," he says as he absentmindedly stabs at his mashed potatoes, "there are days when I can't even imagine living that long."

The smile is sardonic, and given Jim's attitude lately the words are troubling.

Plowing ahead with his lecture on conditioning, Chris continues, "Look at Nolan Ryan. He took excellent care of himself and pitched until he was almost fifty including his seventh no-hitter when he was forty-four. At the end of every game when his teammates were throwing down beers, he was on a stationary bike. He once said that the key to his long career was that he never allowed himself to get out of shape.

"Same with Cal Ripken—he has a full-sized gym in his house. He credits stretching, proper nutrition, and moderation to his record-setting streak of consecutive games played. Compare those guys with athletes like Mickey Mantle and Joe Namath. Only nine times in thirteen years as a pro was Namath healthy enough to play more than six games in a season. Here's a hint why: he used to say that he liked his Johnnie Walker, red, and his women, blond. And, had Mantle taken better care of himself, he would have been the best ballplayer ever. Period."

Typically missing the point, Troy can only say, "Stretching is a waste of time—you're either flexible or you're not. And all this working out crap is just a bunch of narcissistic bullshit."

"Come see me in thirty years," I say to Troy. "You'll be amazed at how much flexibility and muscle strength you lose with age."

"Hey, Doc. I got a question," mumbles Lou. "My knee hurts like hell right after we play, but is fine a day or two later. What's up with that? And, also, my heel feels like someone took a hammer to it. Do you think it's my shoes?"

"Speaking of feet," pipes in Troy, "my right foot feels like a nail is shooting up through the bottom of the arch. Someone told me it might be *Planter's Itis*, or something like that. Ever hear of it?"

"What a bunch of sorry-ass wimps," interrupts Ted. "My abs are rock hard. A solid six-pack. And, look here," he says while flexing his right bicep, "pure steel—the ladies love it!"

"Well, I got you beat," laughs Lou. "I got me a keg under this shirt. A full kegger, not a wimpy pony-keg, like McGregor!" He bellows and I wince.

Lou continues, "And as far as exercise goes, I remember once when I was out of Camels and the roads were covered with snow and ice, I actually had to walk to the corner store. So, I know about exercise. And, oh, yeah, at the same time, I also picked up a twelve-pack of Bud, a jar of peanuts, a bag of chips, and a package of Ding Dongs. So, I know all about weight-lifting, too." He smiles adding, "A day without Ding Dongs, smokes, and a brewski, now, that's a scary thought!"

Chris shakes his head, "What a bunch of morons. Keep chugging your beer and stuffing down greasy potato chips! *Planter's Itis*—that's great. Idiots, I'm surrounded by idiots! God, help me. You guys are hopeless. Strokes and heart attacks just waiting to happen."

"Whoa, Hoss," says Lou. "Is your thong too tight? You're even nastier than usual. What? Mommy not home when you called last night?"

"Sorry," Chris says softly.

"An apology!" says Ted. "He is human, after all! Hey, don't scare me, Doc. You start going soft, and you'll mess me all up. Who will I find to hate, loathe, and despise?"

"I missed my run this morning," says Chris, the venom coming back in his voice. "My whole day is screwed up when I don't get my run in. If I let that happen on a regular basis, I'll lose my tone and become just as physically pathetic as the rest of you. Now *that's* a scary thought!"

"He's back!" cheers Lou. "Att'a boy, Doc."

Given Chris' mood, I decide not to ask him about the pain in my throwing arm and my nagging low-back pain. Better to just suck in my "pony-keg," and gut it out—so to speak. Just like my dad used to tell me, "Never show weakness, Son, never show weakness." That's what he used to say.

"Hey, Tommy-Boy, you gonna eat those fries?" asks Lou as he reaches across the table. Nothing wrong with his ability to stretch.

What Would Mickey Say?
About Muscles, Feet, Joints, Exercise, and Common Sense

Tom: After Ted Williams lost the batting crown to you on the last day of the 1956 season, he's quoted as saying, "If I could run like Mantle I'd hit .400 every year!" Others have said that if you stayed healthy, you could have been the greatest ballplayer, ever. How does that talk make you feel?

Mickey: First of all, in my opinion, Ted Williams was the greatest ballplayer who ever lived. He was a pure hitter. I was always swinging for the fences, but guys like Williams and Musial had more than just physical ability. They concentrated on making contact and getting on base. I may have had some talent, but those guys were students of the game.

As for all the talk about my injuries and how good I might have been, it makes me feel kinda bad and sad at the same time. I feel like I blew my God-given ability by not taking care of myself. Even that first year, back in the 1951 World Series when I blew my knee out chasing down the ball DiMaggio caught in right-center, I didn't listen to the doctor. He gave me all kinds of exercises to do over the winter, but I never did them. Too much work, I guess. At least, that's how I always felt about rehab. As a result, I would never completely heel before going out again. More than anything, I hated to sit out a game. So, I would play hurt and just make matters worse. In my eighteen seasons there were only three years when I got through the entire schedule without an injury. I had fifteen fractures, injuries, or surgeries that kept me out of games. Shoot, I was never good with investments, but if I had bought stock in a medical tape company back in the early sixties I would have retired a wealthy man. People used to talk about how courageous I was for playing hurt. Hell, I did it to myself. The courageous thing would have been to do what I was told and take care of my body.

Tom: How about weights, did you do any lifting?

Mickey: I really don't want to sound like a smart-ass but the only lifting I did was with a bottle of beer or a glass of booze. Like I said, God gave me a lot of natural ability and strength, and I blew it.

Tom: Any advice for weekend warriors and kids?

Mickey: Well, you gotta keep your body in shape if you want to enjoy sports, or anything else for that matter. That don't mean you have to run ten miles every day or live at the gym pumping iron. Just use your head and pay attention to what your body tries to tell you. Look at some of the pictures of me swinging a bat back toward the end of my career and you will see how bad it hurt sometimes. I loved playing the game of baseball. In fact, I loved all games—baseball, football, basketball, and golf—all of them. But playing hurt wasn't much fun at all. Besides the pain, I knew I wasn't doing my best, and that made everything hurt even more.

Tom: How bad was the ostyomelonitis that developed after you were kicked in the shin in high school?

Mickey: Honestly, it never really bothered me after that first year in high school, but it was really touch and go for a while. If it wasn't for my mom, they would have cut off my leg and I never would have had the chance to play professional baseball. Thank God for penicillin.

Also, most people don't know about this, but the ostyomelonitis threatened my career in another way back in 1951. You see, ostyomelonitis is a funny kind of condition that really never goes away. At any rate, the Army felt it was enough of a risk to classify me as a 4-F during the Korean War. In fact, it was an automatic exclusion from any of the armed forces at that time. But, you see, it was pretty hard for the general public to understand why a kid who could run like the wind and hit a ball a mile couldn't wear a uniform and fight for Uncle Sam. If players like Willie Mays, Whitey Ford, Don Newcombe, Don Larsen, Curt Simmons, and Whitey Herzog could go into the Army, then why not this kid from

Oklahoma? Hell, the great Ted Williams took time off to serve in both WWII and the Korean War, and he wasn't the only one!

Well, the comments I heard from the stands kinda bothered me, but I got used to it. But, one day in Cleveland, I got a letter from some guy who said his son had a bad leg and bad eyes but got drafted anyway and died in the war. He called me a draft dodger and said he was going to shoot me in both of my knees. The letter said he had a rifle with a high-powered scope and that it was going to happen soon. I had no choice but to turn it over to the FBI. Nothing happened, but it sure made me nervous. I tried to get Billy Martin to wear my uniform and play centerfield but he wouldn't go for it. It wasn't just the fans, neither. One columnist wrote: "...What's the big deal? He [Mantle] doesn't have to kick anyone in Korea!"

Tom: If you were playing today, with all we know now about exercise and nutrition, do you think you would have played better? Maybe finished with a lifetime average above 300?

Mickey: Don't take me wrong, buddy, but I'm tired of thinking about stuff like that. Heck, I don't know, maybe. I just don't know. If my head was still messed up, I don't know if fewer injuries would have made a difference or not. Logically, the answer's yes, but who knows. I always thought that 1956, when I won the triple crown batting .353 with fifty-two home runs and 130 RBI, should have been my standard and not my peak; heck, I was just twenty-four years old. I should have had a whole career with those kind of numbers.

The point is, I didn't do the things that I knew I should have been doing. I didn't follow common sense. All I wanted to do was party and play baseball, nothing else mattered and I paid the price.

Tom: What's different about how today's athletes train compared to your day?

Mickey: Well, for one thing, like you said, trainers know a whole lot more today than they did when I was playing. Nowadays, you walk into a training room and they have all this fancy equipment to help speed recovery. Also, nutrition is better and guys tend to keep in shape all year instead of letting their bodies go to hell between seasons. Treadmills, nautilus equipment, and all kinds of machines make it possible to train the whole body. We just didn't have all that stuff when I was playing.

Tom: How did you stay in shape during the off-season?

Mickey: Aren't you paying attention, Tom? I told you. Nothing. I didn't do anything to keep in shape between seasons. I guess the closest thing to exercise was when Billy and I would go hunting. We used to take off quick as squirrels whenever hunting season came around.

Hey, speaking of hunting, I got a story Lou would like. One day, Billy I and decided to take a long drive and do a little hunting on a ranch that belonged to a buddy of mine. When we get there, I go inside to say hi to this guy while Billy stays in the pickup. While he was talking to me, the rancher says, "Mickey, do me a favor. I have an old mule that's gone blind and I don't have the heart to get rid of him. Would you shoot him for me?" I tell him that's too bad, but, sure, I'll be glad to do it for him. So, as I'm walking back to the truck, I figure this would be the perfect time to play a practical joke on Billy—we were always pulling jokes on each other. Anyway, when I get back to the truck, I slam the door and tell Billy, I can't believe it, we drove all the way down here and now he won't let us go hunting on his ranch! I'll show him! I'm going in that barn over there and shoot one of his mules! So, I get out of the truck, go over to the barn and put down the blind mule. When I come back out I see Billy standing outside the pick-up holding a smoking rifle. Billy says, "Mick, I showed that old so and so, too. I shot a couple of his cows!"

The Professor Speaks
About Muscles, Feet, Joints, Exercise, and Common Sense

Tom: Professor? You heard these guys complaining about their injuries and you heard Mickey talking about his lack of conditioning. What do you have to say?

Professor Edwards: Now we're talking about my favorite subject—exercise, or, more to the point, physical activity. Better yet, let's think of it as "body maintenance."

If we just think of the body as a machine, like a car, we'd realize that it requires the right kind of fuel and a certain amount of care and maintenance to keep it running properly. When it rolls off the assembly line, the car is clean, shiny, and working great. If we follow the manufacturer's guidelines, we can expect continued good performance and many, many miles before it's ready for the scrap heap.

Recently, I was in a cab going to the airport when I noticed the odometer. It read 298,095 miles. That's right, almost 300,000 miles! I mentioned it to the driver and he said, "Yep, with highway driving and regular oil changes, there's no reason why it won't last another 50,000 miles, maybe more. We have a back-up cab with 330,000 miles, and it seems to be going strong."

Curious to find out the documented record for most miles on a car, I checked the Internet and discovered Irv Gordon from East Patchogue, New York. In 1966, Irv bought a shiny, new, red Volvo P1800S at the Volvoville dealership in Massapequa, N.Y. On March 27, 2003, as he drove through Times Square as part of Volvo's seventy-fifth anniversary celebration, his odometer read 100,000—for the twentieth time. I'll do the math for you, that's 2,000,000 miles!

In a world where the average car is scrapped after nine years, according to the AAA auto club, and where most owners of vintage cars keep them in storage saving them for collectors' shows, parades, and other special occasions, Mr. Gordon's Volvo P1800S is an anomaly. It has been in continual, heavy use for thirty-six years.

After all those years and some two million miles, Mr. Gordon is practically part of his car, his car is practically a part of him. "If I wasn't comfortable in this car, I wouldn't have taken it all the places it's been," he said.

And it's been to a lot of places—to all of the contiguous forty-eight states as well as seven foreign countries: Canada, Mexico, and five nations in Europe. (A British Volvo dealer flew the car across the Atlantic for an auto show.) Mr. Gordon and his P1800S have survived two accidents: it was rear-ended on the Long Island Expressway, and once, on Interstate 80 in Pennsylvania, a tractor-trailer accidentally latched onto the front bumper of the parked Volvo, inadvertently towing it several miles—with Mr. Gordon inside—until the truck went over a bump and the car was dislodged.

The secret to automotive longevity is routine maintenance, he said. "Most people don't take good care of their cars, but they expect a lot from them."

Mr. Gordon, however, takes meticulous care of his Volvo. The paint gleams and all the moving parts are well lubricated. He has the oil changed every 3,000 to 3,500 miles, the spark plugs replaced every 20,000 ("it takes fifteen minutes to do that") and the carburetors rebuilt every 900,000 miles ("whether they need it or not"). He inspects the brakes and transmission himself, and periodically examines all the hoses, belts, and fluid levels. "I look for bubbles in hoses and anything that is showing signs of deterioration," he said. "It's easy."

The engine is spotless, like a show car's. Unlike a show car, the Volvo is kept outside. His garage is for his two "antique" cars, implying that the '66 has not achieved the status of his '29 Packard and '49 Crosley.

How much of the car is original? The fenders and headlights, destroyed in the accidents, have been replaced. The engine was rebuilt in 1978, when the Volvo reached 680,000 miles. The fuel pump was replaced at 1.6 million. That's about it.

As for whether the P1800S will make it to three million, Mr. Gordon frames it as a question not for the car, but for himself. "By then, I'll be getting Social Security," he said. "I'll be lucky to have my teeth and all my hair."

Tom: So, Chris was right when he told us that with regular exercise, stretching, and proper diet, there's no reason why we can't be active into old age.

Professor Edwards: Absolutely! Let's take a look at what Irv said about his old Volvo and apply it to us. For some reason, Tom, we expect that this body of ours will simply take care of itself, no matter what we do to it. If you'll let me play with the car analogy, it's like leaving the showroom in a brand new Vet, Porsche, or—if you like to get places on two wheels instead of four—a Harley Road King Classic and expecting that the vehicle will always perform the way it did when you drove it home.

Now, every new vehicle comes with an owner's manual, right? It's a booklet telling you what to do to keep it running smoothly and dependably for years to come. Usually, the manual will have sections on general maintenance, scheduled maintenance, where to go for service, and even a section on do-it-yourself maintenance. Some manuals will also have a section dealing with how you can tell if your vehicle needs attention.

Well, years ago, just for fun, I took a vehicle manual and substituted body, mind, and spirit where it mentioned the vehicle. I was going to turn it into a book, but just never got around to it. I brought it with me. Let's see now, it's here some-where in my backpack. Yes, here's the basic outline…

MAINTENANCE REQUIREMENTS

Your vehicle (body) has been designed to have fewer maintenance require-ments with longer service intervals to save both your time and money. However, each regular maintenance (physician checkup) as well as day-to-day care (personal lifestyle) is more important than ever before to ensure smooth, trouble-free, safe, and economical driving (living).

It is the owner's responsibility to make sure the specified maintenance, including general maintenance services, are performed (it's up to you). Note that both the new vehicle and emission control system warranties specify that proper maintenance and care must be performed (all guarantees for a life of fulfillment are off if you don't take care of yourself).

General Maintenance

General maintenance items are those day-to-day care practices that are important to your vehicle (body) for proper operation. Again, it is the owner's responsibility (not Mom's, Dad's, Uncle Fred's, your wife's, your sister's, brother's, or cousin Louie's) to ensure that the general maintenance items are performed regularly. These checks or inspections (examinations) can be done either by yourself or your dealer (physician).

Scheduled Maintenance

The scheduled maintenance items listed in the "Owner's Manual Supplement/ Maintenance Schedule" are those required to be serviced at regular intervals.

It is recommended that maintenance and any replacement parts used for maintenance or for the repair of your vehicle (body) be dealer-supplied (stay away from quacks).

The owner may elect to use maintenance services and non-dealer-supplied parts for maintenance and part replacement purposes without invalidating the warranty. However, use of parts and services, which are not of equivalent quality, may shorten the life and impair the effectiveness of the vehicle (your life).

Where to Go for Service

Your authorized vehicle technicians (licensed healthcare practitioners) are well-trained specialists and keep up to date with the latest service (health) information through technician bulletins (medical journals), service tips (physician consults), and in-dealership training programs (continuing medical education seminars). They are well informed about the operation of all the systems on your vehicle (body).

Be sure to keep a copy of the repair order for any service performed on your vehicle (keep good medical records).

What About Do-It-Yourself Maintenance?

Many of the maintenance items are easy to do yourself, if you have a little mechanical ability (common sense) and a few basic automotive tools (guidance and support).

Tom: Okay, okay, I get the idea. We probably need a manual for living that is just as clear-cut as a manual for our cars, but isn't that a little simplistic? We're a lot more complex than a car or a motorcycle. Life just isn't that easy.

Professor Edwards: I don't know, Tom. Sometimes I think we make things—life—more difficult and puzzling than it has to be. That goes for all aspects of life, not just what we're talking about now—mainly our physical bodies. It also applies to our mental and spiritual health as well, but more about that later. My guess is that our softball friends and Mickey will give me a chance to talk about health—in total—as the weeks go by.

Tom: Can you really use a car or motorcycle maintenance manual as a model for tracking men's health?

Professor Edwards: Well, you be the judge. I took each of these bullets directly from my own car manual and made some adjustments. First, here are the warning signs for the car:

Does Your Vehicle Need Repairing?
1) Engine missing, stumbling, or pinging
2) Appreciable loss of power
3) Strange engine noises
4) A fluid leak under the vehicle. (Water dripping from the air conditioning after use is normal.)
5) Change in exhaust sound. (This may indicate a dangerous carbon monoxide leak. Drive with windows open and have the exhaust system checked immediately.)
6) Flat-looking tires, excessive tire squeal when cornering, uneven tire wear
7) Vehicle pulls to one side when driving straight on a level road
8) Strange noises related to suspension movement
9) Loss of brake effectiveness, spongy-feeling brake pedal, pedal almost touches floors, vehicle pulls to one side when breaking
10) Engine coolant temperature continually higher than normal.

Tom: Great! I am particularly interested in how you're going to handle symptoms 3–5…

Professor Edwards: Okay, here goes…

1) Engine missing, stumbling, or pinging
Clearly something is wrong, but it's difficult to put your finger on what it might be. Actually, quite often we use engine terms to describe how we feel: "I feel sluggish today," "I don't seem to be hitting on all cylinders," "I'm out of

gas," and "I can't seem to keep my motor running," are all expressions we've heard or used ourselves.

While not critical, these are symptoms worthy of our attention if they persist. Being "out of sorts" every once in a while is no big deal, but when it becomes more pronounced and seems to show up on a daily basis, it could well be the beginning of something serious, like heart disease.

Symptoms of heart disease vary according to the type of heart disease. Unfortunately, some heart diseases cause no symptoms early in their course. When symptoms occur, they vary from person to person. Symptoms may include chest pain, shortness of breath, weakness and fatigue, palpitations (the sensation of the heart beating in the chest), lightheadedness, and fainting, or feeling like you're going to faint.

Recommended Action:

Like a car engine, it may just be that you got a bad tank of fuel or that you need to take your body out on the road and clear out the lines. If it is periodic, look for a physical cause and try to avoid what you think may have created the problem. Like Lou, maybe it's the two cheeseburger lunches or the pizza at midnight that makes you feel this way. Or, maybe it's the pitcher of beer after the game that has you feeling foggy and queasy. The bottom line is to *pay attention*. If you're missing, stumbling, and pinging on a regular basis, at a minimum you need a tune-up, so go see your physician. Before long, if left untreated, you may blow a gasket and that can't possibly feel very good. If you're a smoker, you may need a new air filter (and you know what that means…).

Of course, as indicated above, if you are having chest pain, shortness of breath, weakness and fatigue, palpitations, lightheadedness, and fainting, or feeling about to faint, you may be having a heart attack so seek treatment immediately!

2) Appreciable loss of power

We all know the difference between feeling kind of lazy and sluggish and feeling flat-out drained and zapped. This "bone-tired" feeling can mean a number of things, from a signal that you're headed toward a bad cold to something much more serious—up to and including heart disease or cancer. Now, don't jump to conclusions and overreact. Again, I'm not talking about one day out of 100, and I'm not talking about how you feel after sitting on your butt all week and then playing touch football with the kids on Saturday morning. I'm talking about something that is showing up every day. Just like a dirty carburetor will pull power from an engine, a serious infection, a failing heart, or a tumor will pull energy from you. The point is, when it is *appreciable*, you know it. And when it shows up *every day*, you know that as well. Sustained lack of energy will impact every aspect of your life and will not be ignored.

Recommended Action:

If the onset is sudden (your engine just stalls) for no apparent reason, take action sooner than later. Call your doctor, call a nurse, or call the emergency room. If the collapse of strength comes with chest pain, nausea, and pain to other parts of your upper body, neck or head, get attention immediately, it could be a stroke or a heart attack.

If it's progressive and you've noticed a building trend toward less and less energy and strength, call your doctor and see him or her as soon as you can. The cause may be physical or psychological or both. Be honest and let the doctor know *exactly* how you feel. Macho guys may look better in their caskets, but they're still in their caskets…and usually way too soon.

3) Strange engine noises

First of all, whenever you find yourself using the word "strange" or "unusual" to describe a sound your body makes or a feeling you have, it needs your attention. Again, the key words are *chronic* and *acute*. Both signal potential trouble. Chronic means constant and regular, and acute means intense—usually sharp and sudden. *Harry's Hotter Than Hades Chili* washed down with *Sallie's Sassy Sangria* may create strange and unusual sounds and feelings bursting from all parts of your body; however, in this case moderation and common sense might be all the cure you need.

If we think of the "engine" as being your heart, and you describe palpitations in terms of hearing your heart beat, you may be in love, you may be frightened, or you may be having a heart attack or a stroke (see 1 and 2 above). If there are creaks in your neck and cracking sounds in your back, this may suggest that you need a trip to your chiropractor for a simple spinal adjustment, or it may signal something more severe. The important thing is to listen (literally and figuratively) to your body.

Neck pain may result from abnormalities in the soft tissues—the muscles, ligaments, and nerves—as well as in the bones and joints of the spine. The most common causes of neck pain are soft tissue abnormalities due to injury or prolonged wear and tear. In rare cases, infection or tumors may cause neck pain.

In some people, neck problems may be the source of pain in the upper back, shoulders, or arms.

Degenerative diseases that cause neck pain include osteoarthritis and rheumatoid arthritis. Osteoarthritis usually occurs in older people as a result of wear of the joints between the bones in the neck. Rheumatoid arthritis can cause destruction of the joints of the neck. Both of these major types of arthritis can cause stiffness and pain.

Cervical disk degeneration can also cause neck pain. The disk acts as a shock absorber between the bones in the neck. In cervical disk degeneration (typically occurring at age forty and upwards), the normal gelatin-like center of the disk degenerates and the space between the vertebrae narrows. As the disk space narrows, added stress is applied to the joints of the spine causing further wear and degenerative disease. The cervical disk may also protrude and cause pressure on the spinal cord or nerve roots when the rim of the disk weakens. This is known as a herniated cervical disk.

Because the neck is so flexible and because it supports the head, it is extremely vulnerable to injury. Motor vehicle or diving accidents, contact sports, and falls may result in neck injury. The regular use of safety belts in motor vehicles can help to prevent or minimize injury. A "rear-end" automobile collision may result in hyperextension, a backward motion of the neck beyond normal limits, or hyper flexion, a forward motion of the neck beyond normal limits. Most common injuries are to the soft tissues, i.e., muscles and ligaments. Severe injury with fracture or dislocation of the neck may damage the spinal cord and cause paralysis (quadriplegia).

Much less common causes of neck pain include tumors, infections, or congenital abnormalities of the vertebrae.

By the way, take a look a Lou's posture. He tends to slouch and carry his head forward out in front of his body. This will create a considerable amount of strain on the neck and shoulders resulting in headaches, backaches, neck aches, as well as pain across the shoulders. If not now, sooner or later, Lou is going to experience a lot of discomfort.

Recommended Action:

If severe neck pain occurs following an injury (motor vehicle accident, diving accident, fall, or sports injury), a trained professional, such as a paramedic, should immobilize the patient to avoid the risk of further injury and possible paralysis. Medical care should be sought immediately. Immediate medical care should also be sought when an injury causes pain in the neck that radiates down the arms and legs. Radiating pain or numbness in your arms or legs causing weakness in the arms or legs without significant neck pain should also be evaluated.

If there has not been an injury, you should seek medical care when neck pain is continuous and persistent, and severe and characterized by pain that radiates down the arms or legs accompanied by headaches, numbness, tingling, or weakness.

And, one more time, and it won't be the last time...if you have the symptoms of a heart attack as described above, get help immediately! Keep in mind that it isn't just guys who look like Lou who are at risk for heart disease. A very close friend of mine recently suffered a severe heart attack. He is the *last* person whom we would consider "at risk." In fact, he is considered by everyone to be a model of physical fitness. At fifty-three years of age, he plays hockey, runs and walks regularly, uses alcohol moderately, has never smoked, his blood pressure and cholesterol readings are enviable, and he seems to have his stress well under control. His problem? He fell out of the wrong family tree. *Pay attention to family history!*

4) A fluid leak under the vehicle. (However, water dripping from the air conditioning after use is normal.)

Okay, now bear with me here, but this is important, particularly as men get older. And, sorry for the crude analogy, but, hey, it happens. To paraphrase the Bard, *"...a fluid leak by any other name is still a fluid leak."* Well, maybe it was Lou who said that after downing a six-pack of Bud, but you get the idea.

Because women are more likely to develop urinary incontinence, male bladder control issues are often overlooked. Stress incontinence, for instance, is often considered to be a woman's disorder. While male bladder control problems differ somewhat from women's disorders, they cause just as much emotional stress and embarrassment.

Prostate problems are often to blame for urinary incontinence. An enlarged prostate can affect male bladder control since the urethra passes through the prostate gland. When enlarged, the prostate can compress the urethra and prevent the normal flow of urine. The brain receives the message to urinate, but the blockage prevents normal urination. This type of incontinence, called urge incontinence, can be treated in a number of ways, including sticking to a preset bladder-voiding schedule. This prevents too much urine from accumulating in the bladder.

Other prostate problems, especially cancer, can affect continence. Or, more accurately, the surgery required to correct prostate problems can damage the urinary sphincter. Many of the surgical procedures for prostate cancer involve this risk and can sometimes lead to stress incontinence. Symptoms of prostate cancer include both the feeling of an urgent need to urinate as well as an inability to urinate. Problems starting and stopping (dribbling) can also be signs of prostate cancer. And, certainly, blood in the urine and pain during ejaculation are also causes of concern and need physician attention.

While prostate problems are among the most serious causes of male bladder control disorders, other causes exist. Urge incontinence can also be caused by blockages in the bladder itself. Bladder stones can reduce urine flow and are often associated with infections unless treated.

Intense physical activity can cause urinary leakage. Again, this condition is more common in women, but male athletes in high impact sports also suffer from this condition. Sports like football, hockey, and rugby put the body under great physical stress and make extensive use of the abdominal muscles. As these muscles (often very strong among athletes) push down on the bladder, they can force urine through the urinary sphincter valve.

Recommended Action:

Male urinary incontinence occurs primarily in aging males and in the majority of instances is related to diseases of the prostate and/or their treatment. Treatment of prostate disease frequently involves altering the prostate, either by medication or surgery. The malignant prostate (prostate cancer) can also alter bladder emptying, but in this situation treatment of the prostate, such as radiation or surgery, is necessary. Regardless of whether the primary problem is malignant or benign, the alteration of the prostate is significant because the sphincter or control mechanisms are in the same anatomical region. If these are altered in the process of treating the prostate, various degrees of urinary incontinence may occur.

Increased urination and frequently feeling the need to urinate can also be symptomatic of Type II Diabetes, particularly if one or more of these conditions are also present: thirst, increased appetite, fatigue, blurred vision, slow-healing infections, and impotence. See your physician and get tested and treatment, if needed.

A seemingly small but significant tip is to try to keep the bladder from becoming too full. My sense is that, at times, perhaps Lou and Troy are not all that discriminating when it comes to finding "emergency restrooms," but the rest of us guys prefer the indoors whenever possible.

5) Change in exhaust sound. (This may indicate a dangerous carbon monoxide leak. Drive with windows open and have the exhaust system checked immediately.)

Well, this opens more doors than a bellman in Manhattan, but I'll keep my comments focused on the clinical side of the male gastro-intestinal system. Let's begin with belching, heartburn, and "sour" stomach and see where it takes us. By the way, I could just as easily have called this section "Life with Lou."

No matter what you think or how many "Who Can Belch the Loudest" contests you may have won at Roosevelt Elementary School, force, volume, and tone from either end of your body are not signs of masculinity or of good health. In fact, they may indicate serious problems up to and including peptic ulcers, reflux disease, Crohn's disease, irritable bowl syndrome, colitis, Diverticular disease, and colon cancer.

Let me just encourage everyone to, again, pay attention to your body and "listen"—pun intended—to what it's telling you.

If you are constantly reaching for antacids, Imodium, stool softeners, laxatives, anti-nausea medicine, and Beano®, your exhaust system is in bad shape and needs attention. It may be you have a bad tank of gas, or you need to change your grade of oil. Perhaps you have a dirty carburetor or a blocked fuel line. Then again, as in the case of those who hang out with Lou, you may just need a new fan belt and open windows.

Recommended Action:

If your exhaust emissions are noxious, and more spontaneous than planned, your output may be related to your input. Gassy foods produce…you guessed it, gas! Also, cut back on the hot spices, monitor dairy products, watch out for alcohol on an empty stomach, and go easy on the fiber (yes, yes, yes—fiber is good for you, just pay attention…).

Again, let common sense rule. If you have blood in your stool, "backsplash" every time you belch, experience chronic diarrhea, and/or can't keep food down, see your physician.

And, while we're at it, guys need to stop self-medicating for chronic conditions without consulting a physician. Look at a package of Tums, for instance, and it will tell you, *"…do not take more than ten tablets in twenty-four hours and do not use the maximum dosage for more than two weeks."* Yeah, right. I can hear Lou now. Actually, I wish I couldn't, but I can. And, judging by the force, volume, and tone, my guess is that he hasn't lost anything since his good old days back at Roosevelt Elementary.

6) Flat-looking tires, excessive tire squeal when cornering, uneven tire wear

Foot problems can affect everyone during their lifetime. Pain and disability can have a considerable impact on mobility and quality of life. Corns, calluses, Plantar warts, heel pain, "runner's toe," and toenail fungus are common, painful, treatable, and, in most cases, preventable. Aging guys who want to keep playing the games that they learned as kids need to pay particular attention to their feet. Also, keep in mind that a sore foot can lead to a sore ankle, can lead to a sore knee, can lead to a sore hip, can lead to a sore back, can lead to...

Remember when you were a kid and all you had for shoes were a pair of PF Flyers, Saddle Shoes, or Hush Puppies for church? Um, well, okay. Maybe just those of you who were born before Eisenhower was president know what I'm talking about. If you're trying to remember what Eisenhower looked like, close this book and come back when you're older. If the thought of Hush Puppies makes your mouth water for fried catfish, don't even bother coming back when you're older.

At any rate, footwear has come a long way since I was a kid in the 1950s. We now have shoes for pronators, supplenators, tennis players, golfers, walkers, cyclists, and for those who aren't sure what they are, we have cross-trainers! There are shoes for every foot and activity. There are also gel insoles, heel cups, orthotics, and sport-specific socks. So, why so many sore feet?

The answer is good news: we're living longer and staying more active as we age. Bowling, bocci ball, horseshoes, billiards, and shuffle board continue to give way to over-forty softball leagues, cross-country skiing, mountain trekking, adult ice-hockey, masters' swim clubs, race walking, tennis, roller blading, cycling, and jogging. Even golfers are walking more than riding. We are more active, and that's good for our hearts and for our lungs. However, without proper equipment, moderation, time for muscle recovery, and—here it comes, again—common sense, all this activity is not so good on our feet. It's also tough on our joints (particularly knees and hips) and our backs.

Recommended Action:

One of the best things you can do for your feet (legs, ankles, knees, hips, pancreas, liver, heart, trunk, neck, and head) is keep your weight down. Obesity is the leading cause of orthopedic problems.

As mentioned, make sure you are wearing the right shoes. I know it's tempting to dig out whatever you can find in the closet or to use someone's hand-me-downs, but it's worth the extra bucks not to suffer the pain. And, in the long run, it's cheaper as well.

7) Vehicle pulls to one side when driving straight on a level road

Well, now, of course I could be talking about one of our softball boys walking home after a beer (or four) from Frazier's Pub on Packard Road, or I could be cryptically referring to Ted falling off the fidelity wagon while a wonderful wife and baby wait for him at home, but I'm not. In this case, I'm talking about something else. I'm talking about vertigo, dizziness, confusion, and loss of coordination. I'm talking about men and strokes.

Every sixty seconds someone in America has a stroke, and every three-and-a-half minutes someone dies from one. But in 40 percent of all strokes, the body offers a warning sign that can mean the difference between life and death.

That warning sign is a transient ischemic attack (TIA), a temporary deficiency in the blood supply to the brain that comes when plaque deposits and blood clots narrow arteries. TIAs usually last only five to ten minutes. Symptoms include:
- sudden weakness
- tingling or numbness on one side of the body
- vision loss
- difficulty with speech
- headache

While these signs are the same as those of stroke, there's one important difference: in a TIA, the symptoms disappear completely within a few hours, leaving no adverse effects. A stroke, on the other hand, can cause lasting, debilitating damage. We can think of a TIA the same way as we think of chest pain. It's a warning—a blessing—telling us that something is wrong and needs our attention, *now*!

Recommended Action:

Like so many health issues, there are lifestyle factors that impact the likelihood of having a stroke, and surviving if one should occur. For example, getting regular medical checkups, controlling diabetes, high blood pressure and heart disease, not smoking, eating a low-fat diet, keeping the pounds off, and exercising regularly.

On a number of these counts, there is at least one of our ballplayers that I am worried about, Tom. Any guesses?

8) Strange noises related to suspension movement

I hear creaky knees, rusty elbows, cracking toes, and necks that snap, crackle, and pop. Is it a casting call for the Tin Man in *The Wizard of Oz*? Jack LeLane pulling a train with his teeth to celebrate his ninetieth birthday? Or, is it the sound of The Rolling Stones on tour? No, no, and maybe, but...no. It's the sound of the Aging of America. The more we age, the more we try to move, the more noise our bones seem to make.

Of all the bone and joint problems that come with aging and overuse, the knee and the shoulder seem to take the biggest beating, especially the knee, and for good reason.

The knee is the largest joint in the human body and one of the most complex. It allows us to walk and run, execute a variety of different body positions, and change the direction of our body movement. However, the knee also serves as an important focal point for weight bearing. It is subjected to tremendous forces—approximately four times the body's weight during walking, and about eight times the body's weight when running. This, combined with the unique structure of the knee joint, makes knee problems the number one reason people seek the attention of an orthopedic specialist. An estimated four million people seek treatment for knee injuries and pain each year.

The term "overuse injury" refers to the effects of repeated, minor trauma to the knee joint. This trauma may result from recreational or competitive running, or jumping as a sport or as part of a sport, such as in basketball, or in the case of our lunchroom gang, softball. The injury occurs gradually, and symptoms may not interfere with the performance of the activity at first. When symptoms do appear, they are usually noticed within twenty-four hours of performing the activity that is producing trauma to the knee. These symptoms may include a dull ache, a specific type of discomfort when the joint is moved a certain way, such as a burning sensation or shooting pain, and sometimes pain when the affected area is touched or pressure is applied to the leg. Pain may be accompanied by swelling.

Recommended Action:

Resting the joint and using first-aid measures, such as elevation and ice therapy, may bring relief. This goes for shoulders as well as knees. However, you should consult an orthopedic specialist if you cannot change your activities to rest the joint or if symptoms persist. In some cases, your activities can be modified to lessen the trauma on the affected joint, or special equipment may be used to provide additional support to the affected area. The orthopedic specialist can help prevent a recurrent injury by prescribing exercises to improve the strength and mobility of the affected joint and its supporting structures.

While joints are the main source of chronic pain, muscle tears and pulls can be really painful and take days and even weeks to heal. I recommend the old tried and true RICE method:

> **R**est: take a genuine break from strenuous activity until you are sure that the injured area is well on the way to recovery.
>
> **I**ce: cooling the injured area gives not only pain relief, but also helps to reduce inflammation and limits tissue damage by reducing the blood flow to the area.
>
> **C**ompression: limits swelling.
>
> **E**levation: this will drain off the fluid leakage that causes swelling. Try to keep the affected area raised above the level of the heart.

Over-the-counter painkillers, also known as analgesics, can also help to relieve temporary pain after an injury. Some painkillers, such as ibuprofen, also have an anti-inflammatory effect and can help to reduce any swelling that is associated with the injury.

You could also try gentle massage or using heat sprays, rubs or ice packs. Bandages supporting the joint may help too.

As the pain begins to subside, you may restart the activity, but should do so at a lower intensity and duration than normal.

9) Loss of effective braking

If we think of braking as slowing down, resting, or coming to a complete stop, we are looking at both physical and psychological concerns. As mentioned earlier, let's stick with the physical for now. There is no question that these guys will give me ample opportunity to comment on psychological concerns.

Let's take a look at sleep patterns. It is free, requires little or no effort, is available just about anywhere you can rest your head, and, to use another car metaphor, it is the ideal time to recharge your battery, both physically and mentally. There's nothing like a good night's sleep to prepare you to face the day's challenges.

Each year, 85 percent of all Americans experience some form of transient insomnia. Every night, 30 percent of the population either find it difficult to fall asleep or they wake in the middle of the night and can't get back to sleep. About 17 percent of these people consider insomnia a serious disruption in their lives.

There are three types of insomnia:

• Transient
• Short-term
• Long-term

Transient and short-term insomnia result from things like having to give a speech, worrying about an important meeting, beginning a diet or changing your diet, travel, an injury, post-surgery, changes in altitude, or a personal crisis.

Long-term insomnia or chronic insomnia can have adverse physical or psychological effects. Knowing the causes of long-term insomnia is critical. You cannot ignore the inability to find restful sleep. On the physical side of cause, chronic insomnia can be the result of medical disorders like hypertension, Parkinson's disease, reflux disease, and asthma. Substance abuse, tobacco, and alcohol can also disrupt sleep.

Recommended Action:

Exercise and rest go hand in hand. If you want to maximize the benefits of exercise and minimize physical risk, you have to get your sleep—you have to re-energize your body for the next day.

At one time, coaches felt that rest was so important that they told their athletes to stay away from sex the night before a big game—so they wouldn't be "spent" and unable to perform during the game. Of course, it was a bit of a challenge to monitor, and the fact is, a good love life can help a guy sleep better. Now that doesn't mean prowling the bars until three in the morning looking for a sleep mate, like young Troy. It simply means that healthy physical relationships round out the man and help bring peace and rest both day and night. Certainly, we will talk more about relationships later, but it seems to fit in the "Brake" section of our manual, as well.

Here's a classic insomnia fighter you can use—others will follow when we talk about stress:

Progressive Muscle Relaxation—Often, sleep is difficult because of muscle tension. This tension may be so subtle that you can't even detect it. Well, remember the old saying "If you can't beat 'em, join 'em"? Here's a perfect example. Don't fight it; go ahead and let your muscles be tense…but do it systematically! Here's what you do:

Shake out your arms and then your legs. Settle back and take a deep breath. Let your body become heavy and relaxed. Concentrate on relaxing.

Take another deep breath. Close your eyes, and keep them closed for the remainder of this exercise. Take a deep breath before you contract each group of muscles as this exercise progresses.

Tighten the muscles around your eyes and your forehead. Squeeze them tighter and tighter, then relax. Relax your forehead. In your mind's eye, see the tension flow away from your eyes and eyelids. Relax your forehead and eye area completely.

Tighten the muscles of your cheeks, jaw, and neck. Tighten them as tightly as you can, then relax completely.

Continue tightening and relaxing each part of your body in sequence. Don't forget to take a deep breath before you contract each muscle group. Follow this pattern:

Your shoulders

Your arms

Your trunk—chest, abdomen, and back

Your thighs and buttocks

Your legs, calves, and feet

When you are finished, you should be completely relaxed—absolutely free of muscular tension. If you practice progressive muscle relaxation, you will be able to generate the relaxation response more efficiently, more quickly, and in environments where you often feel a great deal of tension.

A few more things: avoid caffeine products—chocolate, coffee, and tea—for at least two hours before bedtime, no water an hour before bedtime, and never, never, never eat pizza with Lou at midnight!

10) Engine coolant temperature continually higher than normal

This one we need to pay attention to in two ways: the obvious body fever warning that occurs with an infection, and the less obvious and increasingly deadly rise in body temperature that comes from heat exhaustion brought on by strenuous exercise, insufficient water, and hot weather conditions.

Heat stroke occurs when the body is unable to regulate its temperature. The body's temperature rises rapidly, the sweating mechanism fails, and the body is unable to cool down. Body temperature may rise to 106°F or higher within ten to fifteen minutes. Heat stroke can cause death or permanent disability if emergency treatment is not provided.

Warning signs of heatstroke vary, but may include the following:

• An extremely high body temperature (above 103°F, taken orally)

• Red, hot, and dry skin (no sweating)

• Rapid, strong pulse

• Throbbing headache

• Dizziness

• Nausea

• Confusion

• Unconsciousness

Recommended Action:

If you see any of these signs, you may be dealing with a life-threatening emergency. Have someone call for immediate medical assistance while you begin cooling the victim. Do the following:

- Get the victim to a shady area.
- Cool the victim rapidly using whatever methods you can. For example, immerse the victim in a tub of cool water, place the person in a cool shower, spray the victim with cool water from a garden hose, sponge the person with cool water, or if the humidity is low, wrap the victim in a cool, wet sheet and fan him or her vigorously.
- Monitor body temperature, and continue cooling efforts until the body temperature drops to 101–102°F.
- If emergency medical personnel are delayed, call the hospital emergency room for further instructions.
- Do not give the victim alcohol to drink.
- Get medical assistance as soon as possible.

Sometimes a victim's muscles will begin to twitch uncontrollably as a result of heatstroke. If this happens, keep the victim from injuring himself, but do not place any object in the mouth and do not give fluids. If there is vomiting, make sure the airway remains open by turning the victim on his or her side.

According to a University of North Carolina study released in 2002, nineteen high school and college football players have died from heatstroke since 1995. A group of sports medicine experts claim that two popular diet aids, ephedrine and creatine, may be to blame for an alarming surge in heat-related deaths among athletes.

Not to go light on the subject, but tell Lou and Troy that beer doesn't count. They need pure water or a fortified sports drink like Gatorade to fend off heatstroke.

OWNER'S MANUAL SUPPLEMENT/MAINTENANCE SCHEDULE

To help ensure that your vehicle (body) operates at peak performance for years to come, follow this recommended maintenance schedule:

Physical Exam:
every three years from age twenty to thirty-nine
every two years from age forty to forty-nine
every year after age fifty (including breast exam)

Blood Pressure:
every year

Tuberculosis:
every five years from age twenty to thirty-nine

Blood and Urine Tests:
every three years from age twenty to thirty-nine
every two years from age forty to forty-nine
every year after age fifty

Electrocardiogram:
every three to five years after age fifty, or after thirty if at high risk for heart attacks

Tetanus Booster:
every ten years

Rectal Exam:
every year after age forty

PSA (Prostate Specific Antigen):
every year after age fifty
if at high risk, every year after age forty

Hemoccult:
every year after age forty

Sigmoidoscopy:
every three to four years after age fifty

Colonoscopy:
at age fifty and every ten years thereafter
if at high risk, a colonoscopy at age forty

chapter
four

Supersize That Order and Throw in Some Extra Salt, Please
Diet and Weight Control in the Village of Someday, the State of Denial

*B*lown *away by the amount of food Lou throws down each day, the lunch crew teases him without mercy. Lou is his good-natured self; however, you can tell that his skin is wearing just a little thin. He talks about how he has always been heavy and hints at the difficulty it caused him growing up.*

Chris uses the opportunity to give a nutrition lecture that, for the most part, falls on deaf ears. It's not the information that bothers the group, it's Chris' condescending way of scolding that drives everyone crazy.

The group starts talking about different types of diets including high-fat and low-carb, low-fat and high-carb, Weight Watchers, Jenny Craig, Slim Fast, etc. Chris, again, tries to take over; however, his suggestions are so rigid nobody pays any attention to him. Celebrities like Dan Goodman, Mama Cass Elliot, Barry White, and Orson Wells show up in the conversation. Inevitably, the weight conversation turns to women and what the "ideal" woman looks like.

True to his character, Lou finds a way to joke about their discussion and deflects the embarrassment that he is feeling.

When lunch ends, Mickey talks about the training tables of athletes past and present. He mentions that, in his day, little regard was given to nutrition. Professor Edwards gives a full run down on the risks and benefits of various diets, the controversy about sodium, and the dangers of obesity, including heart disease, bone and joint problems, and adult-onset Diabetes. The professor also looks at food from a sociological and psychological perspective.

I don't know why, but I'm amazed when I look around the cafeteria and see so many overweight people. Of course, our cafeteria is no different than the mall, church, the movies, or anywhere else. Try it yourself—look around; overweight people are everywhere. Even in my mirror!

The reason is no big mystery. Next time you're at the grocery store, look at the shopping carts around you and you will see lots of junk—high fat, great tasting junk! Well, maybe not in your cart, but in everyone else's.

Today, as I look at my own lunch tray, this is what I see: fried chicken, mashed potatoes with gravy, Jell-O salad, coffee, and apple pie.

Now, I don't need the professor to tell me that my heart probably isn't all that pleased with my selections—particularly with the fried chicken, gravy, and pie. But, hey, listen, I played ball last night; I exercised. And, besides, when I look around and see what others are eating, I don't feel so bad. Compared to Lou's tray, mine looks like a Weight Watchers' special.

"Hey, Lou! Did you leave any for the rest of the plant?" jabs Troy. "Good thing this isn't one of those all-you-can-eat cafeterias. The company would go bust and we'd all lose our jobs. Damn, Big Guy, where do you put it? On second thought, never mind, it's pretty obvious where you put it!"

Chris, between sips of his broccoli soup, adds, "I keep telling you, Lou, one of these days you're going to keel over at lunch and one of us is going to have to give you mouth-to-mouth."

"In other words," Troy quickly adds, "Doc says you're gonna die, 'cause it'll be a frosty day in hell before anyone of us gets near your ugly mug."

Ted pipes in, "Honest to God, Lou, how can you eat so much junk? I'm used to seeing your three cheeseburgers and fries, but TWO cookies, besides? No wonder you got thrown out from right field."

The others smirk, pitch winks, and laugh out loud thinking of Lou chugging down the base path as the right fielder easily throws him out.

"Hey! That was a line shot that even Mantle in his prime couldn't run out. Besides, you see how small these cookies are? Used to be twice this size. So, it's really like only having one. And…they *are* fat-free! In fact, I think I'll get two more!"

Munching on his carrot stick, Chris asks, "Serious question, Lou. Have you always been big?"

"Always."

"*Always?*"

"Always. At least as far back as I can remember and in all the pictures from when I was a kid. I weighed twelve pounds when I was born."

"Your mom and dad, are they big, too?" I ask.

"Dad's skinny as a rail, but Mom could whop anyone in the WWF—she's a great cook, too."

"How about hypertension, Lou? Mom or Dad?" asks Chris

"Both."

"I don't suppose you want to hear my sixty-second lecture on the dangers of high blood pressure, do you, Big Guy?" says Chris.

"Got that right, Lycra Boy, but you can pass me the salt."

Throwing his hands up and looking at the rest of us, Chris grunts, "I give up!"

"'Bout friggin' time," says Lou, as he washes down a colossal bite with a huge gulp of chocolate milk.

Looking left and directly at Lou, Ted says, "My brother was a chunky little kid and was constantly teased. Did you ever get teased, Lou?"

"Yeah, until I beat the crap out of Tommy Cusimano in the fifth grade," answers Lou, without lifting his head. "Nobody dared teased me after that."

Something about his tone said that the subject of the Big Guy and his childhood as a fat kid was now closed.

I ask Ted, "You've got little kids—do you let them eat junk food?"

"McDonald's? Wendy's? Yeah, sometimes. Probably more than we should, but Carol makes them eat their vegetables and gives them vitamins—so it all balances out. I suppose we all eat more than our share of snacks, but like Lou's cookies, Carol buys the fat-free stuff—even potato chips, so it isn't that bad."

Looking like he's going to hit someone, or something, Chris can no longer contain himself. "No wonder obesity is growing at an epidemic rate! Guys, think for a minute, will you? It all boils down to calories. Most fat-free foods still have high levels of sugar, and sugar—if not burned—is stored as fat. Our fleet-footed first-baseman is diluting himself with those cookies." Turning to look directly at Lou, he adds, "The last thing you need are cookies. ANY cookies!" Swinging his head to look at Ted, "And your little kids, Ted, are going to be big, fat kids if you keep feeding them that junk."

I can't resist asking, "So, Chris, what are we supposed to eat? Cardboard and carrots?"

"You know what, guys? Just eat whatever you want, but don't come crying to me when you have your heart attacks and strokes."

In a quieter tone, he adds, "Listen, just be reasonable. Try this for lunch, sometime: one cookie, one lean hamburger—better yet, make that a turkey or chicken sandwich—throw in some fruit and vegetables and you're on the road to recovery. If you seriously want to learn about nutrition, come to one of my classes or stop by the office. We will have you keep a food diary, analyze how you're currently killing yourselves, introduce you to the exercise machines, and make recommendations."

"Hey, Doc," slurps Lou, "I keep a diary, and every night I write in it how blessed we all are because you're in our lives."

"Screw you, Fat Boy."

"Not in this lifetime, you Tofu Twerp."

Sensing that this could get even uglier, I ask Chris, "When's your next class on nutrition? I just might show up. God knows what I'm doing now isn't working."

Turning away from Lou, Chris responds, "First Monday of every month."

"Sign me up! I'll be there," I say with more conviction than I'm actually feeling.

"If you're serving nachos and cheese, sign me up, too!" laughs Lou, as the tension clears.

"How about that pork rind diet?" asks Ted. "You know, the one where you can't eat bread but you can eat all the meat you want? My wife's sister lost thirty pounds eating nothing but chicken, cheese, and hamburger."

Chris nods, "You're talking about the Atkins Diet. High protein, low carbohydrate. Very controversial. In my opinion, it's risky and the jury is still out. Jenny Craig and Weight Watchers are two reasonable approaches to weight loss, but exercise is the critical component. Personally, I'm considering becoming a vegan."

"Well," says Lou, "I'm a Presbyterian, but what's that got to do with anything?"

"No, you dufus," responds Chris, "a vegan is someone who doesn't eat any meat—including chicken and fish. Nothing that once had a mother. And no dairy products, either. No milk, eggs, or cheese."

"So, Tom was right," says Ted. "Cardboard and carrots!"

"Hey, I'm a fat, meat-eating, all-American man and proud of it!" shouts

Lou. "Look at all the famous fat people—Babe Ruth, Jackie Gleason, John Candy, Drew Carey! Not a tree-hugging panty-waisted wuss in the bunch!"

"Yeah," adds Troy, "and how about Chubby Checker, Marlon Brando, Oliver Hardy, Luther Vandross, and The Big Bopper!"

"Orson Wells and Winston Churchill," adds Jim, speaking for the first time today.

"Barry White and Mama Cass," says Ted.

"And," with a voice of finality, says Lou, "let's not forget, Santa Claus, Elvis, John Goodman, Buddha, and the Pillsbury Dough Boy!" He laughs again while patting his rotund belly.

"Okay, okay, wait, wait, wait," interjects Chris, leaning forward, determined to ruin the spirit.

"Mama Cass died of a heart attack in her early thirties and Candy also died from a heart attack when he was in his early forties. I think Oliver Hardy died in his sixties from a stroke. Babe Ruth was a slob and Orson Wells was a drunk *and* a slob! Barry White never saw sixty and Luther Vandross suffered a serious stroke in his early fifties.

"Fat people are not happy, healthy, or productive. They're miserable, sickly, and they cost all of us a ton of money in healthcare! And, it's getting worse. Keep laughing and eating those cheeseburgers right into your grave!"

"Careful, Lycra Boy, your blood pressure's rising."

"Up yours, Butterball."

"Screw you, Doc."

And so ends another lunch.

What Would Mickey Say?
About Diet and Weight Control

Tom: How about diet and weight issues, Mick? Any concerns?

Mickey: Well, I sure put on a lot of weight after I stopped playing ball, but it never really bothered me that much. In fact, when I grew up, fat guys were running things. You know, like it was a sign of success or something. Big gut, big cigar, big caddy, big glass of booze, all that stuff.

In the 1950s and 1960s, we liked our women a little big, too. Not fat like Mama Cass or Kate Smith, but healthy looking, like Marilyn Monroe or Jane

Mansfield. Big hair and big boobs—blond, too, if you're asking.

Girls today look sick and almost scary. When I see one of those skinny little gals with no behind, I want to take her out and buy her a good, thick steak and a baked potato with all the fixin's. Throw in a juicy piece of apple pie while you're at it, the kind with the big sugar crumbs on top. Ah, hell, Tom, now you're making me hungry—put a scoop of vanilla ice cream on top of that pie and make that crust with cheddar cheese baked right in, just like they do at this little diner on Highway 412 east of Tulsa.

Tom: Now you're making me hungry, and we just ate! Did the guys you played with pay much attention to diet and weight?

Mickey: Naw, not really. Oh, they paid attention to food. Lots of it! But weight wasn't much of a problem. Keep in mind, we're talking about "The Show," "The Bigs." Most of the guys I played with were pretty fit just from playing ball. The model for all of us, Babe Ruth, looked like he was out of shape, but he was just built kinda funny—big chest, skinny legs. The Babe was 6' 2" and weighed 215, in his prime. He also stole 123 bases.

Now, Yogi looked like he was fat but, again, he was just built funny, a little short and squat. Well, all right, I guess at 5' 8 and 200 pounds he was a little heavy, but as they say, it was all muscle—well, *almost* all muscle. By the way, people remember all his goofy sayings but forget that he hit .285 for his career with 358 homers. He also won the MVP three times and played in fourteen All-Star games and fourteen World Series. Hell, he even stole about thirty bases during his career. Not bad for a little fat kid from St. Louis.

Remember, the designated hitter didn't start until 1973. Before that every player, including the pitcher, had to be able to run, hit, and throw. You had to be a complete athlete—no lard-butts sitting on the bench got to hit without sweating it out on the field. Hell, today, you can have a millionaire designated hitter swing once, get on base, and go sit down again when the manager sends in a designated runner.

Tom: But you were also a football player—good enough to be offered a scholarship to Oklahoma, right? What do you think when you see today's line-backers weighing 340 pounds and running backs that weight 230?

Mickey: Shoot, Tom, I think what everyone else should think. Bad knees, bad back, bad heart. Maybe not in their peak playing days, but it will catch up with them. Got to. Once I turned forty, my legs ached like crazy and my knees hurt all the time. I was just less than six-foot and weighed about 200 pounds when my body was taking a beating on the field. I can only imagine what hauling around another fifty or 100 pounds would have done.

By the way, do you know what Yogi said to his wife, Carmen, when she said she was taking their son to see *Dr. Zhivago*? "What the hell's the matter with him now?" Also, it's true that, once, when I asked him for the time, he said, "You mean right now?" Honest, to God, Tom. He really said those crazy things.

The Professor Speaks
About Diet and Weight Control

Tom: And you, Professor Edwards? What about men and food, or is it just a women's concern?

Professor Edwards: When you ask about "men and food," Tom, what you're really asking is, "Do men care about how they look?" And the answer is yes, of course they do. What little boy hasn't stood in front of a mirror, sucked in his gut, flexed his muscles, and puffed out his chest?

Women talk about body image and how Barbie dolls and super models create this idealized picture of how a woman should look. They point to eating disorders and damaged self-esteem as the outgrowth of society's pressure to look a certain way. Well, it's no different for men. A lot of little boys cry themselves to sleep because some pretty girl called them fat, and other boys shake in fear on the school bus because bullies use them as punching bags.

Tom, you and I are about the same age. When we were kids, who were our comic book heroes? They were Superman, Batman, Spiderman, and The Green Hornet, right? Remember what was on the inside, back cover of those comic books?

Tom: I sure do. Charles Atlas ads. "Hey Skinny! Yer ribs are showing!" I can still see the picture of the bully kicking sand in the guy's face.

Professor Edwards: That's right! I teach a course on "Men and the Media" at the university and I use those ads in class. I have one here, somewhere. Yup, here it is.

I love this last frame where the girl says, "Oh Joe! You are a real He-Man, after all." And in the background the beach crowd is shouting, "WHAT A MAN!" No more ninety-seven-pound weakling for this guy!

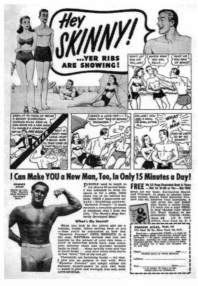

Tom: I'm ashamed to tell you, Professor, but I sure fell for it. I sent in for all that stuff.

Professor Edwards: Don't be ashamed, Tom. All you really wanted was to fit the image that society was telling you was desirable. You wanted to be liked, admired, and successful. And, to do that, you had to have those muscles—or some bully was going to throw sand in your face.

Well, fifty years later, it's really no different. Looks matter. Guys with muscles—*society's definition of handsome and fit*—still get the girls, win the games, sign the contracts, and move up the corporate ladder. Perhaps more to the point, the guys who are too fat (or too thin, too bald, too gray, too old) tend to finish back in the pack. We still equate physical appearance with ability, vitality, sexuality, character, and status. And, honestly, it's hard to imagine that in another fifty years it won't still be the same.

Tom: A bit of a gross generalization, don't you think, Professor?

Professor Edwards: Certainly. But for every Bill Gates or Woody Allen, who make it to the top rungs of their profession, there are 100 Tom Cruises and Arnold Schwarzeneggers already there and another 100 pushing close behind. It's just a fact. And don't think for a moment that men don't feel the body image pressure almost as much as women do. They just don't like to talk about it. They're afraid if they do, someone will kick some more sand in their face.

Tom: Okay, but what about guys like Lou and others who put the weight on and can't, or don't, want to take it off? What happens?

Professor Edwards: Probably nothing new for you here, Tom. It's the same concerns you read about all the time. Carrying extra weight makes your body work harder and can interfere with how your body works internally. If you are overweight, you are more likely to have many health problems, including:

- Raised blood pressure and stroke
- Elevated cholesterol and fat levels in blood (triglyceride) and heart disease
- High blood glucose levels and diabetes mellitus
- Colon and prostate cancers

- Knee and ankle pain and osteoarthritis
- Gallstones
- Sleep apnea
- Hernia
- Sexual difficulties
- Varicose veins

Tom: You're right. I've heard it all before. If you're too fat, you run the risk of heart disease, diabetes, cancer, and problems with your joints. But, what's this about your sex life? Now you have my attention.

Professor Edwards: Certainly, there is the psychological issue of poor self-esteem and a lack of confidence that leads to a less-than-desired sex life. But I'm really talking about impotence—erectile dysfunction or ED, as the clinicians refer to it. Of course, terms like "half-mast," "limp noodle," and the British expression, "Brewer's Droop," is probably more clearly understood by some of the guys at our table. This last one, "Brewer's Droop," aptly describes the unfortunate result of too many cold ones after the game.

Things like smoking, obesity, and alcohol can all impact a man's ability to have an erection. Smoking and obesity impact circulation, and the alcohol is a central nervous system depressant that interferes with the neurological processes necessary for erection. As Shakespeare wrote so insightfully in Macbeth (Act II, Scene 3, line 34), alcohol "provokes the desire, but takes away the performance."

Tom: Okay, but if I can get us back to weight for a moment. I understand it's bad for you to be overweight, and I understand what happens when you're carrying around too much fat. But, listen to what Lou said at the table. He said he's been fat all of his life and it sounds like Mom was too. What can he do about it?

Professor Edwards: Some men are genetically vulnerable to becoming obese, and it sounds like Lou may be one of them. But environment and habits are the biggest influence on your risk of becoming overweight or obese. Ding Dongs, Twinkies, Budweiser, cheeseburgers, apple pie, and chips may have more to do with Lou's super size than his swimming in a fat gene pool.

Tom: But look at Chris. I bet he weighs 200 pounds and he can't be more than six-foot, tops. According to weight tables I've seen, he's at least ten pounds overweight, but he doesn't look like he has an ounce of fat on him. And, how about all those professional athletes? According to those tables, they're all overweight, or even obese!

Professor Edwards: Healthy bodies come in all different shapes and sizes. The Body Mass Index (BMI) is a scale that shows you if your weight is in the healthy range. A healthy weight is BMI between 18.5 and 24.9. [16]

It also matters where your body stores the excess fat. Research has shown that people who have most of their fat stored around their waists/tummies (apple-shaped) will have a higher risk of having heart disease and diabetes than those who carry it around their hips (pear-shaped). Determine your waist circumference by placing a measuring tape snugly around your waist. This risk increases with a waist measurement of over forty inches in men and over thirty-five inches in women.

chapter
five

Just Beneath the Surface...
Stress, Rage, Depression, and Suicide

Quite a week to review. The talk begins with the shiner sported by Troy and his macho re-telling of a mini bar-brawl that ended with Troy spending Thursday night as a guest of The City. Everyone chimes in with their opinion about fights, the movie, Fight Club, *hockey, road rage, little league parents, and violent video games.*

News continues to spread about last weekend's suicide of Jerry Spatalie from engineering, a soft-spoken guy that kept to himself. He left behind a note, a wife, and two pre-teen kids. Speculation runs wild but nobody—at least, none of the men in our group—want to talk much about it.

Jim worked closely with Jerry and he sympathizes with Jerry's decision. He argues that a person should have the right to decide when and how he dies. "Besides," says Jim, "who knows what goes on in a man's life and in his head? We shouldn't judge."

As the chapter closes Mickey talks about bar brawls, violence in sports, his own depression, and thoughts of suicide. Professor Edwards gives a rundown on stress and presents a prescription for a healthy and happy life.

"Well, Troy," I begin, "do you want to tell us about it or should we just wait for the afternoon paper?

"Ouch!" I add after inspecting the bruise under Troy's left eye and the bandage over the right one.

"So, where were you guys?" asks Troy with a sneer. "I turned around and everyone was gone. Thanks a hell of a lot."

"Hey, man, I warned you," says Ted. "I knew if you didn't stop shooting off your big mouth, you were going to get your butt kicked. So what happened?"

"First of all, I didn't get my butt kicked. I did the kicking. And, thanks to you guys, I spent the night in jail."

"No shit…jail?" asks Lou.

"Yeah, jail. Why didn't you guys stay?"

"Wait a minute. Jail? You spent the night *in jail*?" Lou asks again.

"Damn, Lou. Yes! Jail! The Slammer! The Hoosegow! The Can! Disturbing the peace, public intoxication, and assault. My hands hurt like hell—but I won the fight! And it wasn't my fault. Besides, if you think *I* look bad, you should see *them*."

"Troy," says Chris, "I left Annie's at nine o'clock and you were already into your second pitcher. When did this happen?"

"When Lou and I left at eleven o'clock," adds Ted, "you were hitting on every woman in the bar."

"And a couple of the guys, too," laughs Lou trying to break the tension. "We saw the massacre coming, but couldn't get you out of that place. You were one mean son-of-a-bitch. What got into you, boy?"

"Hold on," I say, "did you say, 'them'? Was it those guys from the game?"

"Damn straight. I kicked their tails…with no help from you guys! Come to think of it, I didn't need your help. I didn't need anyone's help."

Turning to his right, Chris says, "Troy, what's up with you? What? You think it's cool that you got in a bar fight and landed in jail? Are you nuts? You could lose your job for a stunt like that or wind up serving time."

"It's no big deal. I don't have any priors and I don't think they'll press the assault charge. They're too embarrassed to admit that I took on three of them and kicked ass!" Troy slams his right fist down on the table hard enough to loosen years of gum wads stuck underneath.

"I expect that I'll have to pay Ernie for damages and that will be that."

"Priors?" says Ted. "Priors? You sound like a cop show. Chris is right, man, this is definitely not cool." Then with a pause, a smile, and a thumbs-up, he says, "Three guys, huh? Awesome! You the Man, Dogg. You the Man!"

Troy gives his best James Dean lip-curl and strokes the bandage above his eye.

Lou asks, "Were you scared?"

"I really don't remember too much—just the rush of adrenaline when I hit that big first-baseman. The one who was lippin' off and making fun of your waddle when you ran down to second base."

"Oh yeah," Lou says with a wince, feeling a distant pain as he thinks again about the Tommy Cusimanos of the world and fifth grade. "So, were you scared?"

"Hell no! It was a rush like I just said. In fact, it felt pretty good. Especially when he went down."

"Was anyone seriously hurt?" I ask.

"No, not really. Cuts, bruises, stuff like that. Mostly, like I said, it's their pride that got hammered."

Ted asks, "Did any of you guys see the movie, *Fight Club*, with Brad Pitt and—what's his name?—Ed Norton? The one where all these guys get together just for the rush of trading punches? Was it like that, Troy? Did you kinda like it?"

"I told you, I don't remember much, but, yeah, it was a rush; I felt a kind of high when it was all over."

"Troy, man, you are nuts," says Ted. "One of these days, you're gonna pick a fight with the wrong person. There are a lot of wackos out there who would just as soon finish the job with a bullet."

"You mean, wackos like Troy?" asks Lou with only a hint of a smile.

"Yeah, just like Troy," says Chris with a shake of his head. "*Exactly* like Troy."

"All right, Chrissie boy. You and me. Now. Outside," says Troy, first with a scowl and then with a nervous laugh.

No one else laughs.

"Fighting is natural," says Lou. "It's part of who we are—as men—in society. Just look at hockey, or pro wrestling. People love it...I love it. It's great!"

"Yeah," says Ted, "I got to admit, there's nothing quite as exciting as being at a hockey game and watching someone drop his gloves." Making a mock megaphone with his hands, Ted booms, "Let's get ready to ruuummmmmmble!"

This time, we all smile.

I add, "I'm telling you, it's never going to change as long as the standard penalty for fighting is five minutes in a box, accompanied by a standing ovation. And, don't think the owners don't hear the cheers. It's money in their pockets. I'm just really concerned about young kids swinging hockey sticks at each other's heads and parents slugging it out in the stands."

As Lou picks up his second bag of fries and downs the last crumbs and grains of salt, he spits out, "Come on, Tommy Boy! You want we should raise a bunch of sissies who can't take a punch? Hell, when I was a kid, we used to trade arm-slugs to see who was toughest. Remember? You always tried to hit the guy right between the muscle and the bone. Hurt like hell, but you always kinda danced and giggled when you found the spot. And then, when he got you back, you laughed through the tears and did some more dancing."

I smile and nod my head as I remember trading punches with my brother, David, wrestling in Tee Leach's den, and the satisfying feeling that comes with throwing a great block and watching someone flip head-over-heals. Damn, those *were* the days!

Okay, I admit it. Although I think it's bad for kids to watch, and it's barbaric, I appreciate a peek at a good fight on HBO or watching a fight break out at a hockey game. Particularly when a player retaliates after continuously getting slashed, grabbed, and slammed hard against the boards. There's something deeply satisfying about identifying with primitive instincts. For a quick moment, it's me who drops the gloves and delivers a good right cross to the bully. And it feels great! Sorry, but there it is.

Lou gets wound up. "You don't even need to go out anymore. You can get all the action in video games—including blood! Some of that stuff is really gross, but a lot of it is pretty cool. Very realistic! They even got 'em for road rage. You get to drive like the NASCAR guys, shoot bad guys, join gangs, and get the chicks! Great game! Awesome graphics!"

"Lou," says Chris as he throws him a bucket of cold water, "grow up. You're almost forty years old, for Christ's sake. Time to put the Gameboy away, *Dude!*"

"Well, L.B., here's the deal. You can let me have my video games or watch me go crazy the next time some tight-ass jerk like you cuts me off as he talks to his mommy on his new cell phone—your choice."

Quickly finding the need to change the subject, I bring up something everyone is thinking about but not saying a word about—Jerry Spatalie's suicide.

"How are Judy and the kids doing?" I ask Jim.

No response.

"Why would someone do that?" Lou asks no one in particular. "I can't imagine blowin' myself away. Christ, the kids must be totally freaked. Someone said he left a note. Anyone know what it said?"

No one looks up; no one says a word.

"Now that I think about it," says Chris, "he was showing classic signs of clinical depression."

"What do mean," Ted asks. "I didn't see anything."

"Well, it was kind of subtle at first, but I noticed that he had lost a lot of weight and he quit coming to the fitness center. He didn't do any exercise outside of work that I knew of, so that means he wasn't eating."

"I guess that means Big Lou is happy as a clam, right?" says Troy, obviously uncomfortable with the subject.

"Nope," says Chris. "Depression can have the opposite effect. For some depressed people, all they do is eat to escape. They end up gaining a ton of weight and feel even worse. Jerry also looked tired and stressed. A couple times, in the hall, last week, I said 'Hi,' and he walked right by like he didn't even see me."

"Hell, Chris," says Lou, who rarely calls Chris by his actual name, "if you knew, why didn't you do something? Talk to him, get him into one of your stress classes, get him to see a shrink—something!"

"Lou, do you know how many guys and women walk around every day looking pissed off, tired, or depressed? If I tried to counsel everyone who was in a funk, that's all I would have time to do.

"Besides," he continues, "most men don't want to talk about that stuff. You've got to be pretty close to someone to tell the difference between clinical depression—real depression—and the blues. There's no way I could know that Jerry was going to do this, no way."

"But, Chris," Ted adds, "I saw him last Friday afternoon, just a few hours before he did it, and he was all smiles and happy. He looked like he just won the lottery! In fact, I remember it because he looked like the cat who swallowed the canary—like he knew something I didn't."

"He probably did," says Chris with a quiet shake of his head. "He probably did."

"Jim," I say, "you worked with Jerry for years—did you see this coming?"

Quiet during lunch and lost in thought, Jim doesn't respond.

"Jim?"

"What?"

"Jerry Spatalie. Did you see this coming?" I ask again.

Looking at his half-eaten lunch, Jim says, "Who knows what goes on in a man's life and in his head. It's his business, how he dies. We shouldn't judge." He pauses. "Maybe he just couldn't take it anymore."

"Take what?" asks Ted. "Was he having trouble at work? At home?"

Stirring his coffee, Jim doesn't hear a word.

What Would Mickey Say?
About Stress, Rage, Depression, and Suicide

Tom: How about it, Mick? They say you could get pretty angry in your day. How did you handle stress?

Mickey: By now, I think it's pretty clear that I didn't handle my stress too well, on or off the field. On the field, I would pout, kick water coolers, throw bats, and cuss. Off the field, I guess it was about the same. When I had a bad day with a bunch of strikeouts, Merlyn had to keep the kids away. She used to say that a bad day at the plate meant a bad night at the plate.

Tom: How about fights? Did you get into scraps like the one Troy had at the bar?

Mickey: No, not really. I can't help but think of Billy Martin when I look at Troy. Billy was a great ballplayer, but it seems people remember him more for his hard drinking, fighting, and partying than for what he did on the field. Billy hit over .250 lifetime and made the All Star Team in 1956, but when people think of Billy, they picture him in a fight, having teammates restrain him, or seeing some umpire toss him out of game. Sure, he had a temper and I guess he had a bit of chip on his shoulder, but he also filled a role for the team. Hell, when Casey thought we were getting lazy or needed a little fire in our bellies he would pull Billy over before a game and tell him to start a fight during the game. Billy's nature didn't need much encouragement, but he also felt it was part of the game and, in particular, part of the Yankee tradition. In many ways he was a lot like a hockey player given the role of "Enforcer." It was part of his job. Of course, not all his fighting took place on field.

Tom: And you?

Mickey: As for me, I really stayed out of fights…don't really know why, but I preferred to play the role of peacemaker than fighter. Sure I got angry, but mostly with myself for playing poorly. Like I said, kicking things and punching water coolers was my release. I remember once, after missing an outside fastball, I came back to the dugout, threw my helmet, knocked over some bats, and kicked the water cooler. Casey just looked up and quietly reminded me that it wasn't the water cooler that was striking me out.

Tom: Sounds like you got pretty moody at times, Mick.

Mickey: Not when I was kid and not in the early days of my career. Strange as it may seem, I got moodier as I got more successful. The better I did on the field, the more likely I was to jump at people and act like a prima donna. I loved to play baseball more than anything. Just the pure joy of swinging the bat, running the bases, catching and throwing...if I didn't think about it as a job, I was fine. It was only when I forgot it was just a game that I got in trouble and I would let it bother me.

Tom: How did Merlyn handle your moods?

Mickey: Ah, she just always wanted people to think the best about me, kids included. She was constantly making excuses for me and telling me how great I was. This may sound kind of strange, but the more she did that—treated me nice and made excuses for me—the tougher it was. Not at the moment, but later, because I knew most of the trouble I got into and the bad days at the ballpark were really my fault and nobody else's.

Her being nice and all made me feel even worse, and I probably resented her for it. I sure didn't return the favor. I guess I made it pretty tough for her and the boys. No, actually, I don't have to guess—I *know* I made it tough. And God only knows why she put up with me for all those years.

Tom: How bad did the mood swings get?

Mickey: Tom, when I was playing ball, I just buried my feelings at the ballpark, the bar, or in the arms of some woman. But mostly, it was playing ball that kept me in control—if you can call it being in control. Like I said before, baseball was the most important thing in my life—it always came first. Merlyn and the boys were second. So, it wasn't until after I retired that the mood swings got really bad. Scary-bad, in fact.

Tom: What do you mean, "Scary bad"?

Mickey: Well, this isn't easy to talk about, but after I retired, I realized that without baseball, I was nothing. In fact, I didn't even know what to call myself. I sure wasn't a businessman and I wasn't the coach that I always hoped I would be. I was just some guy that other guys wanted to play golf with and buy drinks for. What kind of life is that?

Tom: Oh, I don't know, Mick. Some guys would think that playing golf all day and having guys buy you drinks was a pretty good life.

Mickey: Well, yeah, that's how I felt too, for awhile. Then it would hit me when some salesman would laugh at one of my jokes, that all of this was really phony. I mean these guys just wanted to have their pictures taken with "The Great Mickey Mantle" so they could go back to Des Moines, or Chicago, or Buffalo, or wherever and show everyone and tell stories.

Tom: And, again, Mick, what's wrong with that? You made these guys feel good—helped them tap into their dreams and their memories of being a kid and playing baseball. I can think of a hell of lot more depressing ways to make a living.

Mickey: The problem, Tom, is that once they went back to their hometowns with their pictures and their stories, I was left with just me. Does that make sense? I mean, they went home and I went off to one more dinner or golf outing, signed one more autograph, and let one more "friend" buy me a drink. And, invariably, every day ended with me either sleeping with some woman I met that day or, worse, getting off an elevator, alone, stumbling down the hall trying to focus enough to see the room number on my key, stepping into a room that looked just like all the other rooms I've been in, pouring one last drink—if I hadn't brought one with me from the bar—and finally passing out.

Some nights, I would cry myself to sleep because I felt so lonely or because I was afraid I was going to die. Some nights I wished I would die and I would cry because I knew I would wake up again in the morning. Man, I was just plain lost. I didn't know what to do. So, I would just do each day the same: drink, tell stories, play golf, look for a pretty lady, and pass out or cry myself to sleep. So, how does that sound, Tom? Pretty glamorous, huh?

Tom: Was it really that bad, Mick? Always?

Mickey: No, not always. Sometimes, I had a great time and felt really good, but the problem was that I couldn't always tell if it was real or just the booze. Like I said, I wasn't sure if they liked *me* or "Mickey Mantle." Hell, I didn't like me so it was hard to figure that somebody else did.

It got worse as I got older and as I drank more. I swear there were times when I wanted to kill myself.

Tom: You mean, you actually considered suicide?

Mickey: Yeah. Back around '93, depression was a regular part of my life. I was paranoid, scared, and just plain miserable. When I lived with Danny and Kay, I used to beg them not to go out some nights. I hated being alone.

Tom: How did you handle it?

Mickey: I drank until the feeling went away.

Tom: How did you eventually conquer the depression?

Mickey: Honestly, I don't think I ever did, Tom. At least, not completely. In fact, it got even worse when I finally went to the Betty Ford Center. Of course, that was a good thing.

Tom: What do you mean?

Mickey: Well, like I said before, I felt really bad when Danny and Kay went to Betty Ford. First, because they didn't tell me they were going and I lost my drinking buddies. But, then, I felt like a bum because I figured it was my fault that they got that bad to begin with. I felt responsible for screwing up so many lives. It was probably at that moment—when I finally started to take responsibility for all the harm I caused—that I truly started to turn things around. I guess that was the day I quit blaming everyone else for my problems.

Tom: And you checked yourself into Betty Ford?

Mickey: Yeah, and at first it was really hard, and the depression got worse.

Tom: How so?

Mickey: Well, they make you face your fears and talk about them. You know, kind of take stock of your life and deal with what's real and what's not. As part of the twelve steps of Alcoholics Anonymous you have to tell your life story to a group. You have to talk about your drinking, what you did, and how it made you feel. You have to confront the reality of what role booze has played in your life and the lives of others around you.

Hearing the words stumble out of me was both good and very depressing. I don't think I ever gave it a whole lot of thought until I heard the tears and stories come dribbling and spiting out of my mouth.

The biggest part of my recovery probably came during grief therapy. I had to write a letter to my dad. Oh, man, Tom, talk about sad. I cried the whole time. I wrote about how I missed him, about my boys, and I cried especially hard when I wrote my dad that I loved him. I never told him that while he was alive and I always regretted it.

Tom: This experience—the Betty Ford Center—must have been very painful.

Mickey: More so than I can explain. But, the more I let the pain out, the better I felt. The more I honestly looked at my life and my feelings, the brighter things looked. Truthfully, if I knew before I went to Betty Ford that being that open would hurt so much, I'm not sure I would have done it, but I'm so glad I did. Those last eighteen months of life were the best I could remember since my days playing catch with Dad and my Grandpa Charlie back in Commerce. I only wish I had done it sooner.

Tom: So, Mick, any advice for guys on how to deal with stress, rage, depression, and suicide?

Mickey: I can tell you how to drag a bunt down the first base line, throw on the run, slide, and swing from both sides of the plate, but when it comes to dealing with those other things, I really don't know what to tell you other than don't kid yourself. Don't think you can drink your problems away or that other people can make you happy. Also, don't blame anyone else if you're feeling bad about something. Odds are you had a role in making yourself miserable and odds are even better that things won't change until you do something about it.

Couple more things: knock off all the macho B.S. and get help when you're feeling real blue. Maybe that means talking to a buddy or going to see your doc. Hell, talk to your dog if it makes you feel better, but don't keep it in because you're too embarrassed or ashamed to let anyone know you're scared. It will only come out in some other way, like booze, or yelling at your kids, or screwing up at work. Besides, everyone's scared about something, at one time or another. It's the guys who admit it and get help that win at this game.

Tom: Anything else?

Mickey: Yeah, tell your dad that you love him, even if he's no longer around. And, while you're at it, give your kids a hug and tell them that you love them too. And, then, back it up with how you live your life.

Tom: Done?

Mickey: Nope. Get rid of guilt. If you've made mistakes, admit them and don't make the same mistakes again. Then, move on and don't look back. But, most of all, figure out a way to love yourself. At the end, I got all the other parts okay, the talking part along with telling and showing my family that I loved them, but I never could quite figure out how to shake this guilt or how to love old Number 7. I was getting close toward the end, but I just ran out of time.

The Professor Speaks
About Stress, Rage, Depression, and Suicide

Tom: Professor, so much is written about stress, and it only seems to be getting worse. What advice do you have for this crew?

Professor Edwards: In recent years the harmful effects caused by a highly stressful lifestyle have been widely pronounced. Heart disease, insomnia, ulcers, sexual dysfunction, hair loss, skin irritations, exhaustion, and cancer are just some of the negative consequences of stress. However, it is also important to remember that the same stress level may also produce accomplishment, inspiration, creativity, opportunity, increased self-esteem, improved physical health, and a sense of fulfillment. In fact, Tom, studies have found that the will and desire to live is dependent upon a certain degree of stress and challenge. Yep, stress can kill all right, but it can also heal.

Tom: So, how can guys get control of the stress in their lives and make it work for them? How do they keep from becoming victims of their stress?

Professor Edwards: One of the ways is by seeking and developing a strong external support system—build a strong network of friends and associates who will listen to your concerns and help you sort through various plans of action. Mickey is right when he advises guys to talk to someone about their concerns, even if it is just the family pet. The point is, you have to express your concerns in some manner before you can begin to make changes.

Our lunchroom team is really a men's therapy group. Of course, they would never think of themselves that way. But, in their own manner, they supply each other with sympathy, understanding, objectivity, knowledge, encouragement, and, when necessary, an all-important kick-in-the-seat-of-the-pants! These guys—all guys—need to develop, cherish, and utilize their external support network.

Tom: That's it? Get a bunch of guys like Lou to give you advice? You must be kidding.

Professor Edwards: Hey, I hear what you're saying, but even guys like Lou have good advice to offer, or, at a minimum, they help you see things from a different perspective. It's obviously important to expand your support system to include professionals whenever possible and to not become unduly dependent upon any one segment. The loss of a dominant source of support can be devastating. That's why, in the end, the single most important predictor for mental stability is a well-developed, internal support system accented by balance.

Tom: Wait, Doc. You're starting to get too technical. What do you mean by internal support and balance?

Professor Edwards: Fair enough. I'll try to keep it simple. I agree that some academics try to make this stuff way more complex than it needs to be.

What I mean, Tom, is that our friends, family, business associates, church and civic affiliations are all critically important; however, ultimate happiness and personal accomplishment require that the primary source of support needs to come from within the individual.

If we have a perception—that may or may not be consistent with reality— that all of our external support systems have failed us, it is our internal system that will determine if stress is going to be destructive or productive. In Mickey's case, he became too dependent upon baseball, adoring fans, alcohol, and Merlyn's tolerance. They replaced a solid sense and appreciation of self—a knowing and liking of Mickey by Mickey.

Tom: Wait, Doc. You're starting to lose me again. Are you saying that Mickey felt he was worthless without baseball, and once baseball was gone, he hid in the bottle rather than face his fears and guilt?

Professor Edwards: You're getting there, Tom. In Mickey's case, it probably goes back to his relationship with his dad and an ongoing quest for approval, but that's for a whole other discussion. Basically, you've got the gist of it. Once the pinstripes came off, the headlines stopped, and the girls moved on to younger stars, Mickey had to face troubling issues and he had to face them alone. He didn't have the strength or the tools to deal with what he found.

The strength and the tools for shaping and dealing with life is what I refer to as our *Internal Support System*.

Our internal support system simply determines how we react to stressful situations. Destructive reactions include such things as smoking, abusing alcohol and prescription medicines, using illegal drugs, and engaging in reckless and compulsive eating and sexual behaviors. An internal support system based upon these behaviors is transitory, artificial, repressive, and deadly.

Tom: Okay, so if all of those reactions to stress suggest a poor internal support system and predict disaster, what are we supposed to do when we're feeling too much stress?

Professor Edwards: Productive reactions to stressful situations result in a reduction of anxiety, increased energy, and new opportunities for personal and professional growth. Instead of kicking water coolers or picking fights in bars, practice the following:

Gather the Facts. When you are faced with a stressful situation or you need to make a tough decision, step back for a minute. Then, gather all the facts you need to objectively analyze the problem or make the decision. Don't act impulsively—reserve judgment and action until you have all the pertinent information. If you don't take a minute to gather the facts, your judgments may be distorted, causing confusion and wasted energy.

Assess and Assume Accountability. Mickey's recovery didn't begin until he took full responsibility for his actions. Recognize your role in creating potentially distressful situations. Constantly blaming others will eventually alienate you from your friends, family, and co-workers. With the right tools, you have a great degree of control over how you react to a stressful situation. However, refusing to accept accountability suggests that you do not have control over your life and this lack of control makes you vulnerable to distress.

Make a Plan and Do Something. You can waste time with fruitless dreaming and energy-draining complaining, or you can design a plan and take action. Whether you're solving a complicated work problem or simply deciding what to do this weekend, gather your facts and then make a plan of action. Tackle a large problem one step at a time. Of course, planning alone is not enough—after you decide what to do, you must follow through, or all your talk is just hot air!

Achieve and Maintain Physical Fitness. Exercise and good nutrition are as close to a panacea as we can come. Improved self-esteem, a healthy respiratory and circulatory system, enhanced career opportunities, weight control, and longevity are just a sampling of the by-products of a regular regime of exercise and proper nutrition.

Maintain Perspective. It is important to give each event an appropriate amount of weight and importance. What seems like an earth-shattering crisis today may just be a small hitch in your plans when reviewed tomorrow. As you deal with stressors, try to look at the whole picture. In the total scope of things, what significance should be placed on the event or circumstance? Is it truly devastating? Is there zero hope for the future? There are always conditions for which we can be grateful and new opportunities that we can discover.

Tom: That's it? Respond to life in those five ways and happiness is yours?

Professor Edwards: Well, you can certainly make life as complex as you wish, but it really boils down to how we respond to our environment. That's the only part that we can really control.

The most important thing to remember is that when it comes to stress reactions, we have a choice. One choice is to react in a negative fashion and suffer the consequences. Or, we can learn the facts, appropriately accept responsibility, be active rather than passive, maintain our health, and keep things in perspective. Those five guidelines and a life of balance are about as close as you can get to a prescription for healthy and productive living.

Tom: That brings me back to my earlier question. You answered the first part about internal support systems, but what about balance? What exactly do you mean when you talk about a life accented by balance?

Professor Edwards: Again, let's not make this complicated. It's not. All I mean by balance is that we give an appropriate amount of attention to our bodies, minds, and spirits. It's as simple as one, two, three.

Take care of your body by living a life with no tobacco, little or no alcohol, plenty of rest, good nutrition, manageable stress, low body fat, muscle flexibility, and exercise that is both aerobic and anaerobic.

Stimulate your mind with life-long learning that includes art, literature, music, history, philosophy, and the acquisition of new skills.

Develop your spiritual being through the worship, exploration, and wonder of forces more powerful, compassionate, awesome, forgiving, and knowledgeable than anything you can possibly experience in the physical world.

Tom: And you call that easy?

Professor Edwards: No. I said it was simple. Only you can determine whether or not life is easy, challenging, or impossible. And, guess what, Tom? No matter what you believe, you are correct.

Tom: I'm sorry, what?

Professor Edwards: Never mind, Tom, just a little more psychobabble to keep you thinking. And, here's some more: just because I said it was simple doesn't mean it's not complex.

Tom: No. Please, stop, please. My head is starting to hurt!

Professor Edwards: Just this closing thought on life and stress and I'll let you go. We've spoken a lot about stress and how we respond to it, but we haven't said much about anger, depression, or suicide.

All of us know people who have seemingly been through it all but somehow always wear a smile, offer support to others, and look for good things to happen in the future. In the face of hardship, tragedy, disappointment, a demanding workload, and family responsibilities, they not only survive, they thrive! Why? How come they don't break? And why is it that other people, with seemingly everything going their way, can't cope with even life's small, everyday challenges?

The reason is that while the solution steps are simple and straightforward, implementation and compliance is a highly complex blend of psychology, physiology, sociology, and, in some cases, pharmacology.

Rage, depression, and suicide are all subjective reactions. Divorce, illness, accidents, and other seemingly cruel and random life events, settle on points along a continuum that has Ultimate Pain on one end and Ultimate Pleasure on the other. Where we place ourselves determines our level of pain or pleasure. Let me say that again. *Where we place ourselves determines our level of pain or pleasure.*

No matter what you may think, adults are not tossed, bullied, or forced toward either end of this spectrum. We may not always have a choice when it comes to life events, but we do have a choice when it comes to how we respond. And it's our response that determines the level of pain or pleasure we experience.

Absent this core belief—that we have the potential to control our lives—we are forever vulnerable to feeling victimized and impotent, with little hope of sustained personal growth and penetrating happiness.

chapter .
six

I'd Walk a Mile for a Camel...But, I Don't Think I Can Make It
The Power and Devastation of Addiction

Although against the company's non-smoking policy, Lou manages to sneak a smoke or two while working on the loading dock. Of course, the guys at the table can smell the smoke and hear his hacking, but rarely make any comments. Today, however, fresh off last week's discussion of Jerry Spatalie's death, Ted suggests that Lou's nicotine habit is just another form of suicide. This leads to an animated discussion of cigarettes, cigars, and chewing tobacco (Lou also chews).

I lost my father and mother to smoking-related disease. Troy never smoked but, as we know, he has his share of addictions. Ted typifies the reaction of a never-smoker, and Chris is uncharacteristically sensitive to the challenges of quitting.

Mickey talks about the role of tobacco in the sports culture and the many tobacco commercials he and other athletes did in the fifties and sixties. The professor talks about how urges are formed and what to do to avoid losing control.

Sounding like a diesel engine starting up on a cold winter morning, Lou clears his throat as he approaches the table and begins his ritual pre-lunch smoker's cough.

"Hey, Lou," Troy says, "that's disgusting! Why is it that every day you hack your lungs out at the lunch table? We're trying to eat here!"

"I think I'm getting a cold," says Lou.

"You always have that cough, Lou," adds Ted. "It's from those cancer sticks of yours. I think we should start a pool to see who can guess what will get Lou first—the Camels or the cheeseburgers."

"I don't smoke that much, anymore," Lou says. "Besides, I'm gonna quit."

"Lou," says Chris, "do you have any idea how many times you've said that? Don't kid yourself, my friend, you'd smoke a French fry if you could. I don't know which is worse, breathing your smoke or watching you spit tobacco all over the ball field."

"Hey! What's with this pick-on-Lou crap? I just sat down. Ease up for Christ's sake!"

"It's because we love ya, Big Guy," adds Troy.

"Well, a little less love, okay? You don't hear me harping about your blood-shot eyes or Lycra Boy's broccoli breath, do ya?"

"You know, I can't remember seeing my dad without a Chesterfield," I tell the group.

"My whole house smoked—all of us," I continue. "Dad got lung cancer when I was in junior high school and he still smoked—we all did. Eventually, his arteries started to break down and they had to amputate a toe, a foot, one leg, and finally the other leg. He died a very painful death. But, we all kept right on smoking even when my mom was diagnosed with emphysema."

"Damn, Tom," says Lou. "How did you quit?"

"I went to a quit-smoking class and never looked back."

"Never?"

"Well, no, actually, that's not true," I confess. "It wasn't easy, but I really wanted to quit, and all the things they taught us about nutrition and stress made it easier. Lots of valuable techniques, too—things to do when the urge struck. But, like I said, the most important part was that I really wanted to quit."

"Actually," says Chris, "most people who quit smoking do it on their own. They just quit. But, Tom's right—it's easier with a program. When you're ready, Big Guy, come on down and see me. As soon as we get enough people interested, we'll schedule another class."

"Yeah," says Lou, "I will—someday—not just now. But, someday. Soon."

The whole time Ted is just shaking his head. "What's the big deal with quitting smoking? Read the label. It says, 'This stuff is gonna kill you!' What else do you need to know? Here ya go, Lou," he continues, "you don't want to smoke, anymore? Then, don't buy 'em and don't bum 'em!

"Next problem, please," says Ted, as he brushes his hands together signifying that the problem is solved.

"Thanks, Ted," says Lou sardonically. "Now, here's some advice for you. Mind your own friggin' business. And, pass the salt."

"Okay, Big Guy, but keep in mind that suicide comes in all shapes and sizes."

Given the open wound left by Jerry's death, the comment about suicide stings everyone. No one responds.

I ask Chris, "How many smokers do we have here at the plant?"

"Our last survey showed about 150 smokers—approximately 30 percent. More than our share."

"How many people show up for your quit-smoking program?"

"Not many. We've got hardcore smokers. According to our last survey, only half of them said they want to quit—just like Lou—but they never show up for classes—just like Lou.

"Some try the patch or chew the gum, but they expect to magically wake up the next day and not want to smoke. Everyone wants a quick fix. When they realize it takes work, they cave in and smoke within just a few weeks. I'd like to help, but I'm running out of ideas."

"It's just will power, that's all it is," says Ted, sounding bored.

"Did you ever smoke, Mr. I-gotta-down-a-six-pack-of-Heineken-every-night?" responds Lou.

Ted shakes his head.

"Well, then don't be so quick to judge."

"I don't drink that much," adds Ted quickly.

"Yeah, right. And, Troy, here, doesn't smoke dope," says Chris.

Without looking up, Troy gives Chris his customary salute.

"Speaking of 'smoke,' it's time to visit the Cowboy for my second dessert," says Lou as he pushes himself away from the table and heads for the shipping dock. Some days he gets in back-to-back Marlboro Lights before clocking back in.

"By the way," I ask, "has anyone seen Jim today, or yesterday?"

They all shake their heads no.

What Would Mickey Say?
About Tobacco and Addiction

Tom: So, Mick, did you ever smoke?

Mickey: Oh, every once in awhile I'd have a cigar and I tried chew when I was a kid, but, no, tobacco wasn't my thing, even though I was a spokesman for Viceroy cigarettes in 1957. But, everyone was endorsing cigarettes back then. Roger was the big smoker on our team. I can't remember seeing Maris without a Camel sticking out of his mouth.

Tom: Roger Maris?

Mickey: Yeah. But he wasn't the only one. We had so many guys smoking in the dugout that Dizzy Dean, Pee Wee, and the guys from TV's "Game of the Week" finally had to ask us to move away from the steps so the kids wouldn't see all the smoke. Dizzy said it looked like the Wabash Cannonball was coming right through our dugout!

Tom: Any advice about smoking and tobacco use?

Mickey: Well, I think the obvious advice is: don't do it! But, my guess is that Professor Edwards, there, will say that it isn't quite that easy.

The other advice I would give is to those who think that change is easy. It isn't. I knew that I shouldn't drink as much as I did and I'm sure that smokers know they shouldn't smoke. The problem is that just knowing something doesn't make it happen. My guess is that if people would be less judgmental and more compassionate, it would be easier for folks to make changes. Like the Indians use to say, "Walk a mile in my moccasins, before you judge me." Or, something like that. You get the idea.

Tom: Well, what about the chewing tobacco?

Mickey: Same thing. Don't do it. I remember Nellie Fox and some of those boys who stuffed so much Red Man into their cheeks they looked like chipmunks. And more than one pitcher swallowed a big ol' plug while dodging a line drive hit back at his head.

I guess it was kind of disgusting, but nobody ever said it was bad for you. Heck, growing up in Oklahoma in the 30s and 40s, there were spittoons in every bar and probably in every parlor, too.

They say it's even more addictive than smoking and can cause all kinds of cancers in your mouth and on your tongue. Even so, I knew guys who tried to kick it but just couldn't. Some of them got off the sauce and stayed off but said tobacco was tougher.

Tom: Anything more to say about tobacco, Mick?

Mickey: Nope. I always wanted to be a coach, and a good coach knows to let his assistants handle the stuff they know best and to defer to them. I would no more try to tell Whitey how to throw a curve ball than he would tell me how to hit a high outside fastball. I'll let the professor talk about tobacco.

The Professor Speaks
About Tobacco and Addiction

Tom: With all the warnings and talk about tobacco, why are guys like Lou still smoking and chewing tobacco?

Professor Edwards: Tom, sit back while I give you both the short answer and the details. There are plenty of places like the Heart Association and the American Cancer Society where you can get good programs and in-depth information about what happens to your body, but I'll let them do that. I am much more interested in following up on what Mickey said about the fact that knowing something does not make it happen. In other words, like you just asked: why does someone do something they know is harmful, stupid, or both?

Tom: How about the short answer?

Professor Edwards: Well, the short answer probably won't be that short, but hang in there because it applies to way more than just tobacco use.

Mickey is right. People often think that stopping or controlling behaviors like smoking is relatively easy. Like Ted said, with smoking all you have to do is read the side of the pack to know that smoking is harmful, then it's a matter of not buying or bumming cigarettes.

Simple, right? Well, of course not. Quitting tobacco is no simpler than losing weight and keeping it off or starting and staying with an exercise program. In fact, because of that complex blend of social, psychological, phys-ical, and pharmacological factors mentioned earlier, tobacco addiction is very powerful. Like Mickey said, some people find it easier to stop drinking than to kick nicotine. In fact, laboratory studies put nicotine in the same category of addictions as cocaine and heroin.

Also, Mickey was right when he guessed that if people were a little less judgmental and a bit more compassionate, it might be easier for people to make lasting lifestyle changes.

With that in mind, here are a couple of examples of what I mean:

Mary

Mary is pregnant and she goes to see her physician. The physician says, "Mary, you're pregnant! That's wonderful! After all these years of trying; I'm so happy for you! But, Mary, I see cigarettes in your purse. Please tell me that they do not belong to you. Right? You're not still smoking, are you Mary? Because if you are, Mary, have you thought of all the complications associated with smoking and pregnancy? Have you thought about how sick that baby is going to be because of your smoking? Have you thought about who is going to take care of your baby because of all the potential problems associated with your smoking? In fact, Mary, given your heart condition and your age, have you thought about WHO IS GOING TO RAISE YOUR BABY? BECAUSE, IF YOU CONTINUE TO SMOKE, YOU WON'T BE AROUND TO SEE YOUR BABY GROW UP!"

Bob

Bob, a heart patient, sees his physician for a regularly scheduled post-surgical visit. The physician says:

"Bob, you are our poster boy for by-pass surgery! Everything went so well, and your recovery appears to be way ahead of schedule. Oh, but Bob...I must have neglected to caution you about passive smoke because I can smell cigarette smoke on your clothes. So, make sure you avoid smoke as much as you can. Bob? Please don't tell me that you're smoking. Huh? After everything you went through, you mean to tell me that you're smoking again? What's the matter with you? Six weeks ago you were on the sixth floor with your chest opened and now you're smoking again! Hey, listen, Bob, did you have a nice Christmas last year? Lots of presents and family gathered together? Tell me, Bob, did they take a lot of pictures of you? Because, if you continue to smoke, that was the last Christmas with your family or anyone else. Next Christmas, YOU WON'T BE AROUND TO BE IN THE PICTURES, BOB! DO I MAKE MYSELF CLEAR?"

Now, Tom, you tell me, what do Mary and Bob do as soon as they leave their physicians' offices? Of course, they light up! They have just been flooded with feelings of guilt, anger, fear, and confusion. All of these emotions are triggers associated with smoking cigarettes, compulsive eating, alcohol abuse, drug abuse, etc.

Keep what Mickey said in mind. Information wrapped in compassion and unconditional acceptance of the person (not their behavior) will go much farther than threats and coercion. REMEMBER: There's a person behind the cigarette, the drink, the cupcakes, the crack cocaine, the...

Tom: And, the more detailed explanation?

Professor Edwards: Let's go back to the pleasure vs. pain continuum that I discussed after last week's lunch, and take a closer look.

Educators often label behaviors like smoking, excessive alcohol consumption, compulsive gambling, compulsive eating, etc. as a "negative coping mechanism." Unfortunately, these behaviors are initiated due to a lack of positive or neutral options for dealing with situations perceived by the individual as threatening or painful. The threat may be either physical or psychological, ranging in intensity from uncomfortable to life threatening.

It is important, however, to point out that the individual assigns a positive value to the tools used to combat the threat. Intellectually, smoking, drinking, gambling, or compulsive eating may be harmful, but the emotional perception is that the behavior is not only helpful, it is absolutely the right road to move the person away from pain and toward pleasure. In other words, intellectually, the person seeking assistance may be 100 percent committed to change, but emotionally they scream for things to remain exactly like they are. Logic, intelligence, family, and personal safety, be damned.

So, why do people continue to engage in actions they recognize as harmful? Are they operating under a death wish? Are they attempting to punish themselves for past evil deeds?

No.

The truth is that these behaviors are more reactive than active. Smoking, excessive drinking, drug abuse, compulsive eating, etc., are reactions to fear, frustration, anxiety, physical discomfort, anger, among other emotions. Unfortunately, psychological addiction occurs when problem resolution and diminished symptoms of discomfort are associated with a specific behavior response.

The anxious worker who retreats into a bottle each night to "resolve" the frustrations of the day begins to establish drinking as the primary vehicle for blocking out conditions that threaten his psychological well being—those things that cause him pain.

The same thing occurs with compulsive eating for stress reduction. Initially, the pleasure associated with tasting favorite foods masks discomfort. This reinforces eating as a problem-solving technique to the point where food, in general, is sought out in response to emotional states such as anxiety, depression, and boredom.

Once a specific behavior response has been assigned a positive value, there is a natural tendency to repeat the behavior whenever the individual perceives threat or pain. The result is the entrenchment of a psychological addiction that is very difficult to break.

In addition to the psychological dependency, there are often intense physical adjustments necessary after such things as quitting the habitual use of tobacco or alcohol, and over consumption of favorite foods.

Part of the difficulty with cessation or control has to do with the associations that trigger desires to return to sworn-off behaviors. Associations can be visual, auditory, tactile, or olfactory, and they can be consciously recognized or unconsciously processed. They are generally transitory cues that historically preceded the behavior that the individual is attempting to control or eliminate. A song, a routine situation, a change in emotional status, aromas, etc., are often associations that cue a desire to relinquish control. It's important to remember that their power belongs to the moment, and if appropriate techniques are applied early, full control will once again belong to the individual. However, if measures for diffusing the power of the associations are employed, the individual will find himself in the middle of a full-blown urge to "fall of the wagon." The power of the urge has such emotional strength that the individual compulsively forgoes all of his resolution in favor of an action from which he is intellectually divorced, but emotionally soldered.

Tom: Where do these urges come from? Do they just suddenly sneak up and capture you at a weak moment?

Professor Edwards: It is important to realize that the desire to forego rational decisions in favor of emotional reactions is developmental. There is a process that takes an individual from being very comfortable with a decision, to desperately wanting to behave as if the decision had never been made. The initial phase of this process is called the *Association Phase.*

An association is any thought concerning the behavior that the individual is attempting to control or eliminate. The thought may be immediately uncomfortable, or the thought may present itself as being very benign, or even helpful (such as thinking how proud the person is because he has initiated the change). The danger comes from the seemingly harmless thoughts. If left alone, however, these harmless reflections will quickly advance to the *Crisis Phase* and then on to the *Obsessive Phase*.

Here, Tom, look at this graph:

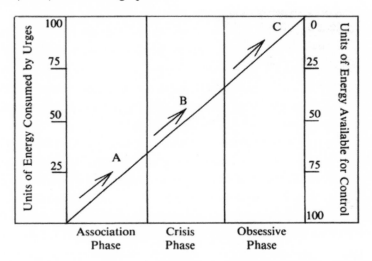

As more and more energy is consumed by the urge, the individual drains his ability to resist compulsive behavior. During the Association Phase, the individual is exposed to a cue (visual, auditory, tactile, or olfactory) that historically triggers the behavior in question. Point "A" on the diagram indicates that an association occurred that initiated thoughts of the old behavior. Given a total of 100 units of energy these thoughts are absorbing approximately 25 percent of the individual's total available energy. With 75 percent of the resources still intact, this would be an ideal time to employ techniques for eliminating the urge. If techniques are not used, the urge will grow quickly into the Crisis Phase. Point "B" shows available energy split between urges and control. If the momentum isn't stopped here, the individual will find himself being catapulted into the Obsessive Phase, which will, in turn, lead him back to the undesirable behavior. Point "C" indicates 95 percent of the available energy is being consumed by the urges—impulsive behavior is inevitable.

Tom, as the diagram suggests, intervention during the Association Phase is a person's best bet for self-control. Available energy is at its highest. However, associations are not always consciously recognized. The individual may suddenly find himself in the middle of the Crisis Phase without any knowledge of how he got there. If that occurs, the individual should concern himself with eliminating the urge, and then retrace the chain of events that led to the discomfort. Once the source of the urge has been identified, measures can be taken to either avoid or control that situation in the future.

Tom: All that makes sense, but how do you keep the urges from growing and taking control?

Professor Edwards: At both conscious and subconscious levels, we can process several bits of information simultaneously. What occurs is that as information is received it is categorized (physical or emotional), assigned a value (good, bad, or neutral), and prioritized for response according to perceived need (immediate or delayed). When an association triggers a thought of a behavior that is in the process of being controlled or eliminated, that thought quickly receives a high priority for response. Once designated for immediate response, the thought will persist until action is taken. *The longer the delay, the more intense the urge.* The individual has two choices for removing the urge—give in to the behavior or initiate control techniques.

The following techniques are among the many effective tools for regaining and maintaining control over obsessive thoughts and compulsive behaviors:

1. **Now Awareness**. The "Now Awareness" technique is designed to distract urges and desires for unwanted behaviors while new behavior patterns are being formed. Remember, an urge is simply *concentrated energy*. If the individual can circumvent that energy—if he can interrupt the flow of the energy—the result will be a lessening of the power of that urge. This, in turn, will allow him to regain control. "Now Awareness" is accomplished by shifting attention from the behavior in question to any physical object in the person's immediate environment. Once the object is spotted, the person should say to himself, "I am now aware of _____," and fill in the name of the object he is looking at. For example, if the person is sitting at his desk when the thought appears, he could say to himself, "I am now aware of the phone on my desk; I am now aware of the lamp on my desk; I am now aware of the pencil," etc. This moves the undesirable thought from a primary position in the conscious mind to a secondary position. Lowering the energy level reduces the likelihood that he will give in to the urge. In addition, because of the transitory nature of urges, the delay caused by "Now Awareness" will allow the urge to pass. Any time an association is met by control, the association is weakened and the opportunity for urges to develop is diminished.

2. **Thought Stoppage**. The objective here is the same as "Now Awareness." We are looking to circumvent the urge, to interrupt the flow of energy. To make

this technique effective, the individual must practice yelling the word "stop" at least ten times so that he can simply close his eyes and hear the sound of the word "stop." The energy level of the word "stop" will override the existing undesirable urge. Initially, it will override it long enough to allow the individual to draw from other techniques. Eventually, the power of this technique will be sufficient to deal with the urge all by itself.

3. **Reminder Wrist Band**. The wristband is another effective way of breaking the momentum of a building urge. By pulling back on the wrist band (elastic or rubber) and letting go in response to an urge, the person is in fact punishing the urge. Quite simply, if "A" results in "B," and "B" is painful, it will not take the individual long to figure out that to remove "B," one first needs to remove "A."

4. **Exercise.** Exercise is another excellent way of diverting an urge. In addition to the psychological lift that comes with exercise, there is mounting evidence suggesting that bio-chemical reactions during exercise naturally produce a state of relaxation. A trip to the physician is advisable for individuals over thirty-five who have not exercised regularly in the past, and for individuals who have a history of cardio-pulmonary dysfunction.

Additional aids for maintaining control include deep breathing exercises, imagery exercises, and basic problem-solving techniques (identification, planning, and implementation).

The previous diagram demonstrated what can occur when an urge goes unchecked. The diagram below shows how urges can be brought under control when intervention techniques are applied.

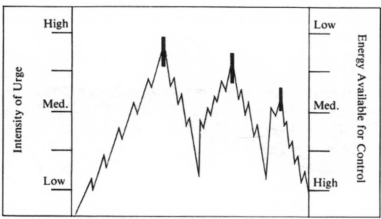

|= Intervention Technique

Tom: I've heard that a person's confidence makes all the difference in the world. How does that work?

Professor Edwards: Now you're talking about what I consider to be the most powerful force in human behavior: Self-Fulfilling Prophecy (SFP). SFP occurs when an individual believes something strongly enough (and that something is within the realm of possibility) to act in a manner that ensures that his belief becomes a reality. A great deal of behavior is directed by perceptions of future conditions. Unfortunately, perceptions generally fall way short of capabilities. In fact, failure to recognize potential often results in negative outcomes.

Why do people engage in prophecies (expectations, perceptions, etc.) that fall short of their capabilities? For one reason, prophecies of failure allow individuals to avoid risk situations. A person who engages in negative self-fulfilling prophecies might approach behavior management (e.g., smoking cessation) in the following manner: "If I try, I may fail—so I won't try." Or, "If I don't try, I can't fail; I may not succeed, but at least I won't fail—so, I won't try." Thus, perceptions of future negative conditions are directing his behavior. This approach to life may result in temporary avoidance of risk, but it also precludes growth and realization of human potential. Let's take a closer look at the work and phrase selection of this individual: "won't," "fail," "don't," "can't," etc. Success cannot breathe in such an atmosphere of negativity.

Tom: Doesn't that also come from other people telling you that you can't do something and that you will fail?

Professor Edwards: Yes. Negative self-fulfilling prophecies are also the result of low expectations by others. Individuals should be aware of people who continually suggest that the outcome of their efforts will be failure. People who project failure for others are often gauging their own status based on the successes and failures of others. The more other people fail, the higher their perception of themselves.

By refusing to entertain such words as "failure," "can't," "won't," etc., and by rejecting low expectations predicted by others, people can use the power of SFP to grow and experience the successes in life that meet their true capabilities.

chapter
seven

Hey, Susie, Did You Hear the One About…?

Sexual Harassment and Misogyny

*T*ed *celebrated last night's softball victory with a blatant display of infidelity and utter disrespect for women. Hitting on every woman at Annie's Dugout, he eventually convinced an obviously impaired—and very young—lady to leave the bar with him. Jim missed his second game in a row, and Chris left for home after a quick beer.*

After watching Ted in action, I thought about his family and started to feel very sad. As quickly as the shortstop and the teeny-bopper snuck out of the bar— yes, they actually crouched down, made ssshhhing sounds with forefingers intersecting their lips, and peeked over their shoulders as they giggled out the door— I lost the after-glow of going 3 for 4. Suddenly, feeling very old, I limped out the door, pointed my minivan toward home, and longed to hug Laurie, talk about mundane stuff, and kiss my kids goodnight.

For weeks, I've kept my mouth shut and even contributed to Ted's behavior by making flippant comments and laughing at his sexist jokes. But, today I can't keep quiet any longer. My sudden case of righteousness spills over and I attack Troy, who, although single and understandably flirtatious, has no more respect for women than does Ted. His chauvinistic contempt is obvious. He views sex and women in much the same fashion as he approaches softball or any other recreation. His goal in life is to have as much fun as possible and damn the consequences to himself or anyone else.

Chris may have his faults, but he appears to be a solid husband and father. He supports my indignation and gives a short lecture on sexually-transmitted diseases. Lou, in character, just wants to laugh off everything.

Jim's a no-show for the third time this week.

Mickey shares a recurring childhood sexual trauma and how it may have influenced his adult relationships with women. The Professor picks up on the theme of childhood trauma and subsequent adult male behavior.

Ted was performing at the table by the time I sat down.

"God was finished making the earth and was speaking to Adam. 'Hey God!' says Adam. 'Looking after all these animals is all cool and everything, but I think I'd like someone more like myself to be with.' God replies, 'Well, I could make you the perfect companion who would be with you all the time, would be faithful, and would never leave your side. But, it'll cost you an arm and a leg.' Adam stops and thinks for a while, and says 'Well...what can I get for a rib?'"

As the table groans and giggles, he continues, missing the irony of his own joke. "Wait, wait, here's another one: Why are hangovers better than women?...Hangovers will go away."

Troy's turn. "What's worse than a male chauvinist pig?...A woman that won't do what she's told!"

Lou adds, "I got one. If your wife and a lawyer were drowning, and you had to move fast, what would you do...lunch or a movie?"

"Hey, Sally," shouts Ted, as our office manager walks by, "I have a question for you. If a man speaks in the forest, and there isn't a woman around to hear him...is he *still* wrong?'"

Sally's tight smile, rolling eyes, and the shake of her head say more than Ted sees.

"Nice, very nice. Yes, indeed...very nice," says Ted, giving Sally an obscene head-to-toe, toe-to-head scan as she passes well within the sound of his voice. "Definitely. Would if I could..."

"Dream on, lover boy," says Troy. "She's way too good for you. In fact, you pinch her fanny one more time and she's gonna bust you."

"She loves it," says Ted with a wink and a bite of his apple. "They all love it. They just want you to think they don't."

Unable to keep quiet any longer, I speak up. "So, how are Lucy and your two little ones these days, Ted? Got any new pictures of the girls?"

Catching my meaning, Ted looks away, slowly nods his head and says, "Fine, just fine, Tom. My wife and children are just fine."

"Great, and did you have a nice time last night, Ted? With your...*celebration?*" I ask, with a tinge of anger in my voice and a steady stare. Each second I think about those little girls and Lucy, the angrier I get.

Everyone at the table looks at Ted. "What's your point, Tom?" asks Ted. "I don't need any lectures from you. What I do is my business."

"Lighten up, Tommy Boy," says Troy. "A little extra-curricular activity—every now and then—is good for a relationship. Keeps everything fresh and new."

"Okay, I got another one," says Lou, wanting to break the tension. "What's the difference between a dead dog in the road and a dead lawyer in the road?...There are skid marks in front of the dog."

It works, but only for a moment.

"Let me tell you," Troy starts back, stabbing the air with his finger, "women are no different than guys. They take whatever they can and leave you hanging. They're out for themselves no matter what you do or how nice you try to be. They say one thing, and mean something else—they make promises one day and break them the next. I believe in the four Fs: find 'em, feel 'em, fuck 'em, and forget 'em!"

"Ouch! Sounds like someone got dumped," remarks Lou.

"At least I have dates, Big Guy! When's the last time you took out a woman? Or, maybe you're more interested in the tall, dark, and bearded ones. The kind with hairy knuckles and a bobbing Adam's apple?

"Here's another one for you, Lou," Troy continues, as Lou shakes his bologna sandwich at him. "What do you call a lesbian Eskimo?...A Klondike."

Lou puts down his sandwich and, in spite of himself, laughs.

As for me, the temptation to leave the table is almost overwhelming. Chris is right—this is a table of morons. I feel like it's 1962 and I'm back at Tappen Junior High School.

Then, surprisingly, Chris comes to the rescue. "So, tell me, guys," he slowly looks around the table, "other than cheating on your women, telling sexist jokes, and sharpening your homophobic humor, what are you doing with your lives?"

Ted ignores Chris and comes back at me, "Tom, how long you been married—this time?"

"Twenty-five years."

"And, never once in those twenty-five years have you screwed around—not once?"

"Believe it or not, no. That doesn't mean that I haven't been tempted or even come close, but, no, I haven't screwed around."

"I don't believe it," says Troy. "My old man was a sales rep and had a woman in every major city in this country. My mom didn't have a clue. Or, at least, she refused to see the clues that she had right in front of her. Finally, one day, he just walked out. I think he actually wanted to get caught so she would throw him out instead."

"I adore my wife and kid," says Chris. "I can't imagine doing anything to hurt them. They're my whole world."

"How long you been married, Chris?" asks Ted.

"Three years, in March."

"Give it time," says Ted. "Give it time. Soon, you'll be singing a different tune."

"Are you guys really this cynical?" I ask. "With attitudes like yours, no wonder you think so poorly of women and relationships. Trust me, it doesn't have to be like that. And, remind me to keep you away from my daughters."

"Okay, enough," says Ted, holding up his hands in surrender. "We're slime balls and we know it. Now, can we leave this conversation?"

"Speak for yourself, slime ball," says Troy. "As for me, I'm just havin' fun while I'm young and free!"

"You may be young, but you're not free," says Chris, again showing unexpected insight. "And, one more thing, keep in mind that every woman you sleep with, you're also sleeping with every man she ever slept with."

"What the hell does that mean?" asks Lou. "That doesn't make any sense."

"Lou, Daddy is trying to tell us that when we go digging in the muck, we gotta watch out for bugs. Ain't that right, Papa Chris?"

"Laugh if you want, but each time you have sex you're looking at the possibility of multiple diseases, including HIV."

"Not if you pick your women carefully and wear a rain coat," says Troy with a smirk.

"Dream on, Romeo, dream on," says Chris, shaking his head.

"All right, new subject," says Ted. "What's up with Jim? He's missed the last two ball games and this is the third day this week he's been out."

"All I know is that he has a flock of sick days coming to him, and he's starting to use them up," I say, giving out more information than I really should have.

What Would Mickey Say?
About Sexual Harassment and Misogyny

Tom: Mickey? What about you and women?

Mickey: I guess I liked women just fine. In fact, Merlyn would say that I liked them too much.

Tom: Your affairs and one-nighters are pretty well known, Mick, but it's also well known that you were often crude and insulting to women. Any comment?

Mickey: This is also real hard to talk about, so bear with me. First of all, keep in mind that it was a different time when I was coming up in the fifties. There wasn't any of the women's rights stuff and, like I said earlier, a guy was judged by other guys based upon how he did with the ladies, how well he could hold his liquor, and how good a jock he was. Also, I was from Oklahoma where the man always wore the pants in the family and the women usually stayed in the background. It's no excuse, but part of all that was the times, the way I was raised, and where I came from.

Tom: How about your mother, were you close?

Mickey: My mom loved us—no question—and she was very protective, but she was pretty strict and not what you would call warm and fuzzy. She wasn't big on hugs and sweet talk. But, I knew she loved me.

Tom: How about sisters?

Mickey: I had four brothers, the twins, Ray and Roy, Butch, and my half-brother from my mom's first marriage, Theodore. My mom and dad had my sister, Barbara, and my mom had another daughter, Anna Bea. I got along fine with Barbara, but Anna Bea used to tease me pretty bad when I was a little kid.

Tom: How bad?

Mickey: Pretty bad, Tom. It was a long time ago, but she and her girlfriends would take down my drawers and laugh and mess around with me.

Tom: What do you mean, "mess around?" Did they molest you?

Mickey: Yeah.

Tom: Once? Twice? What?

Mickey: Actually, on and off for a few years, I guess.

Tom: Did you ever tell anyone?

Mickey: Shoot, no. Are you kidding? I was just a little kid and I was scared of what might happen. When I got older, I felt kind of guilty and embarrassed. I never could have told my dad that stuff and I'm not sure how Mom would have taken it, so I just kept quiet. Anna Bea finally moved out and it stopped, but I never did forget about it.

Tom: Did Merlyn ever know about it?

Mickey: Yeah, after I quit drinking I told her one night. She thinks it helps explain why I was messed up with all those affairs, and why I would be kind of crude around women when I was drinking. Like I said before, she was always making excuses for me—no matter what.

Tom: What do you think?

Mickey: I think it's like the professor, there, says. At some point you have to quit blaming other people and accept responsibility for what you do in life. So, yeah, having your half-sister and her friends depants you, laugh, and play with your little pecker can probably leave some pretty bad scars. But, there are guys who go through worse things and don't end up treating women like dirt and having affairs. In the end, it was me who screwed up. I accept responsibility for everything I did. By the way, that means the good things, too, Tom. I treated my mom really good and, for the most part, I was pretty good to Merlyn, too.

The Professor Speaks
About Sexual Harassment and Misogyny

Tom: Is Mickey's reaction typical for men who were molested as children? And how about Ted's philandering and Troy's disrespect for women?

Professor Edwards: There was so much going on at the table today that it's hard to know where to start. Also, having read Tony Castro's excellent book on Mickey, I was aware of the sexual abuse he experienced. However, the answer to your question as to whether or not Mickey's disrespectful treatment of women can be traced to his own abuse is more difficult to answer than you might expect.

Yes, sure, the fact that his sister and her friends abused him could partially account for how he treated women later in life. However, it's important to point out that the lasting impact of sexual abuse—or any other childhood trauma—is dependent upon a number of factors, including personal makeup, family support, community influence, professional intervention, and the passage of time. A difficult childhood is not a life-long sentence of misery, pain, and dysfunction. In fact, many kids springboard from childhood traumas into a life of deep sensitivity, profound insight, and compassionate service to others.

I have great respect for Mickey when he refuses to duck responsibility for his actions. He understands that regardless of what circumstances you find yourself in now, or what it was like when you were a kid, it all boils down to *choice*. At some point, you have to look in the mirror, quit feeling sorry for yourself, and take charge.

As for Ted and Troy, they are today's version of what Mickey was talking about. Ted is puffing out his chest in a misguided display of virility and a sub-culture's dangerous definition of what it means to be a man. Troy is just plain angry. Angry at his dad's behavior and his mom's tolerance. Most of all, he is angry that neither one of them saw the pain it caused him. In particular, he's furious with his mother—and, therefore, all women—because in his mind, a mother's job is to protect her children, and she failed. At this point in his life, his crudeness, cynicism, and self-destructive behavior clearly show that he has zero sense of responsibility, and an equally blank understanding of the consequences of his actions.

Red flags are frantically waving over the heads of both Ted and Troy, but they can neither see them, nor can they hear their sharp snaps.

chapter.
eight

Sunrise, Sunset
Men, Healthcare, and Personal Responsibility

A week of deep reflection has passed since I last sat down at the lunch table. On Monday, senior management found out that Harvey Martin, our founder, board chairman, and president has end-stage colon cancer. It seems that for years he had symptoms but was too busy or too embarrassed to go see the doctor. When he finally did, the cancer had already spread throughout his body. It's only a matter of weeks now, maybe days. The rest of the week has been hectic with little time for more than a cup of soup at my desk. I missed the game last night but see everyone, including Jim, at our regular lunch table today.

Talk centers around Harvey's cancer, men's reluctance to seek help, and the whole prospect of aging, dying, and death. In response to a question from Ted, I talk a bit about couples living with menopause—both kinds.

"So how's the old man?" Lou asks with obvious concern.

Harvey hired Lou directly out of high school and they have always maintained a special relationship. Truth be known, Harvey was a lot like Lou in the boss's younger days—rough along the edges, a bit crude, but always ready with a laugh and a smile. Give Lou a mechanical engineering degree from Michigan Tech, an MBA from Wharton, and a five-million-dollar inheritance and the two are identical.

Putting down my tray, I shake my head. "Not good."

"What is it? What's he got? Cancer?"

As with any small company, news travels fast. Harvey has always been a hands-on leader. Very visible. It's not unusual to see him in the plant, sleeves rolled-up, grease on his shirt, working on a piece of equipment. He loves this place.

"There will be," I say, looking around the table, "a formal bulletin distributed this afternoon, but, yes, he has cancer and it doesn't look good."

"Prostate?" asks Ted.

"Colon."

"Damn," says Lou. "Colon cancer!"

"It's spread to his lungs, his brain, and even to his bones," I continue.

"Oh, man," says Troy. "That's a shock. He was just pestering me about a new server for our monitoring system. He knew more about the technology than I did. Is he going to make it?"

I slowly shake my head. "We can always pray for a miracle, but the cancer has spread to the point where there really isn't much that can be done—other than make him as comfortable as possible."

"Can we visit him? What hospital? When are visiting hours?" asks Lou, obviously shaken by the news.

"He's at home."

"Home?" Lou says confused. "Why isn't he in the hospital?"

Chris joins in, "Lou, where would you rather spend your time, at home or in the hospital?"

"Yeah, but…"

"Lou, he's dying!" says Jim, recently back after his mysterious absence. "It happens to all of us—sooner or later."

Jim has said the words that nobody wanted to hear or say.

Nobody says anything.

Chris breaks the silence, "How long has he known, Tom?"

"He and Jane just found out about ten days ago."

"But he must have had some idea before that—some symptoms?"

"Well, he had lost a lot of weight and Jane said that he finally admitted that he had noticed blood in his stool, periodically, over several months. Sometimes heavy bleeding. A couple weeks ago, Jane found him passed out on the bathroom floor in a pool of blood. She called an ambulance."

"Jeez, guys!" says Ted. "I'm sorry about Harvey, but do we have to talk about this stuff? I'm trying to eat, here. *Damn*."

"That's the problem, Ted," says Chris. "Nobody wants to talk about cancer. Particularly colon cancer. That's why we're going to lose Harvey. Caught early, it's 90 percent curable. Harvey's dying as much from embarrassment and stupid pride as he is from cancer."

"I noticed he was getting skinny," says Lou, "but I thought I had just lost my cheeseburger buddy. I had no idea."

"This is really personal stuff, Tom," adds Troy. "Are you sure Harvey wants you talking about this?"

"Not only does he want me to, he asked me to. He wants everyone to know about this so it won't happen to anyone else." I look at everyone at the table. "The bulletin released this afternoon will cover all this and more. I know because I wrote it and Harvey signed it."

"Well, fine," says Ted. "I am truly sorry, but can we leave this talk before I projectile vomit all over Troy? Why couldn't you just say he was having digestive problems, or a belly ache, or something a little less graphic. Sorry, I don't mean to be insensitive, but I don't need the gory details."

"Ted," says Chris, "when was the last time you had a physical?"

"Easy," says Ted, "high school football, ten years ago. Look at this body, man. I'm a rock. I never get sick."

"Great," says Chris. "So, when's the last time you checked your testicles?"

"Say what? My *testicles*? Here, Doc," says Ted as he grabs his crotch, "you can check out my testicles."

"Seriously, smart guy, when's the last time you checked yourself for testicular cancer?" says Chris with a deadly serious look. "Have you ever?"

"Chris, I'm twenty-eight years old, never been sick, and I feel great."

"Testicular cancer is most common in men from ages fifteen to thirty-five. You, my friend, are at the age when you should check yourself at least every month. Ever hear of Lance Armstrong?" Chris continues, looking at Ted.

"The guy who landed on the moon?" asks Lou.

"No, Lou," says Troy. "The cyclist. You know, the *Tour de France*."

"Yeah," says Ted. "He had cancer, I know, I know."

"What kind of cancer?" Chris asks.

"Well, since we're talking about my gonads, my guess is testicular. Right?"

"Right," adds Chris, "and he was just as macho as you are until one of them swelled up to the size of a grapefruit and he was spitting up blood. He damn near died because of his 'tough-guy' attitude. Now, he goes all around the world talking about testicles and testicular cancer—all types of cancer—and the importance of paying attention to your body."

"Enough with the blood—enough with the lecture! I get your point! I'll check my jewels, and just to make sure they're okay, I'll also find some fine young lady to check them with me. Just kidding, Tom!" he adds quickly, pointing a finger at me and smiling. "Just kidding."

"Tom," says Lou, slurping down his double-mocha milkshake, "you're about Harvey's age. You ever think about death?"

"God. Only you would ask that question," I say, with both a smile and a slight shiver. "Yeah, certainly more now than I did when I was Troy's age or even Ted's age. Ever since I turned fifty a few years ago, I think more about it."

I continue, "My gut's a little bigger, the knees are a little sorer, I'm really stiff after a softball game—things like that give you subtle reminders that you're aging."

"You forgot the part about your hair disappearing," smiles Troy.

"Thanks for the reminder, kid." I smile in return. "You just wait until you're out of puberty, it will happen to you, too."

There's an interesting feel to today's lunch. The bantering is there and the quick insults still fly, but the feeling is one that can only be described as "affectionate." The news about Harvey and the discussion of death draws us closer. Nobody will mention it, and not everyone will recognize it, but it's there.

"So, is it true you lose your sex drive when you get as old as you?" asks Ted.

"Hey," I say quickly, somewhat embarrassed, "let's leave my sex drive out of this."

"No fair, man," says Ted. "If we can talk about my nuggets, we can talk about an old man's sex drive. What about it? Can you still get it up like the old days?"

Interesting how when the discussion deals with men's issues in general, or when we were talking about someone else, it doesn't bother me. However, this line of questioning does. But, Chris is right. Embarrassment and macho pride can be our worst enemies. Guys don't go to doctors, and men, particularly older men, don't talk to women about these issues. So, who better to talk with than other men?

Before I can answer, Chris adds, "Tell you what, Lou, you keep smoking and you'll fly at half-mast, at best. Smoking causes the blood vessels to constrict and without sufficient blood flow—the party's over."

"Time for Viagra!" winks Ted. "Just ask old Bob Dole, he'll set you straight—so to speak."

"Not always," says Chris. "Sometimes emotional issues can cause impotence that even Viagra can't fix."

Lou sees an opening, "Did you hear that they're coming out with a generic version of Viagra?" he asks with a big smile. "They call it 'Fix-a-Flat.'" We moan. "Wait, wait, there's more. What's the difference between Viagra and Niagara? Niagara Falls! One more, one more," he says, bouncing in his seat. "Here's one for Ted. Have you tried the new hot beverage, Viagraccino? One cup and you're up all night!"

Thank God for Lou.

Thinking I've avoided Ted's inquiry about my sex life proves to be just an illusion. He repeats his question. "How about it, old man, can you still get it up like the old days? Is sex just as good on the downside of life?"

Trying not to get too personal, I keep it in the spirit of guy-talk. "I don't hear any complaints from home, if that's what you mean."

Amazed that I can't talk about this without a giggle in my voice, I try to get serious. "To tell you the truth, sex is better now than ever. There's less concern with quantity and more emphasis on quality. The anxiety to perform is gone—there's more give and take…more communication. Everything is much more relaxed. Our whole relationship is better."

"Better?" asks Ted, with a doubting look on his face.

"Yep. Better," I say with confidence and comfort. "*Much* better."

"No problems?" Jim asks, talking for the first time in a long time.

"Well, sure there have been problems; what couple doesn't have problems?" I continue, "Particularly when Laurie started menopause, or, as Archie Bunker would say, 'The Change.' That was really a horrible time for both of us, but we worked through it. Laurie didn't know what was happening to her—she just felt miserable and really moody. Seems like, at times, she hated everybody and everything, including herself and me. I didn't have a clue about what to do or how to act. It was a really difficult period for us—it probably is for most couples our age. Honestly, there were moments when I wasn't sure we would make it."

Jim raises his head, "What did you do?"

"Better living through chemistry," I say, sounding more flippant than I intended. "Laurie saw her gynecologist and she put her on hormone replacement therapy."

"That's all it took?" asks Jim.

"Well, that, a lot of reading on the subject, and many, many hours of honest discussion. It took time and effort, but since then our relationship has never been better. And, to be honest, I was going through my own form of menopause."

"Oh, bullshit, Tom," says Ted. "Men don't go through menopause. That's a bunch of psychobabble crap."

"Actually," says Chris, "there's mounting evidence that men do undergo chemical changes at Tom's age. It affects men both physically and emotionally. Kind of the same way it does women. Some guys get tired, nervous, insecure, irritable, depressed, and they can't sleep. Plus all kinds of strange feelings, including hot flashes and night sweats."

"Nothing that a blond and a Porsche can't fix," chuckles Ted.

Given the proverbial "Mac Truck" opening, I say to Ted, "Actually, Ted, some guys try to fix things with that formula long before they reach my age."

"Speaking of blondes," says Lou, "how can you tell if a blond's been using the computer?…There's white-out on the screen." He chuckles and—once again—we groan.

For a few moments we forget about Harvey and what he and his family must be going through. But only for a few moments….

What Would Mickey Say?
About Men, Healthcare, and Personal Responsibility

Tom: Did you give much thought to your health and getting old, Mick?

Mickey: Like most guys, I guess I lived by the rule of, "No Pain…No Gain," and the belief that only sissies complained. Part of being a man meant that you gut it out and played when you were hurt and went to work when you didn't feel so good. So, when I was still playing ball, I didn't think much about my health or about taking care of myself. I did think about dying, though. You know, what Howard Cosell called "The Mantle Curse."

Tom: You mean about all the Mantle men dying early with Hodgkin's disease?

Mickey: Yeah. Even though I used to joke about it, I got tired of hearing about it. The worst was when Cosell referred to me as "the doomed Yankee slugger playing out his career in the Valley of Death."

Now that I think about it, maybe that's why I never paid much attention to taking care of myself. I figured it wouldn't matter anyhow.

Tom: How about after you retired from baseball? Did you think about death and dying then?

Mickey: Well, yes, I guess. I would have pretty bad panic attacks where I couldn't breath and I would think I was dying. I had them even as a kid, but they got real bad after I retired. I remember one time, I was on a plane to Dallas and I thought I was having a heart attack because the pain in my chest was so bad. I asked the stewardess if there was a doctor on board and she slapped an oxygen mask on my face. When we got to Love Field they had a doctor, a stretcher, and an ambulance waiting for me. It wasn't a heart attack, it was just nerves.

You see, Tom, I was really very shy and uncomfortable around people. I used the booze to help make me feel more comfortable, but the fear of making a mistake or having people reject me was still there. On the ball field, I was just fine as long as I was playing okay. But if I didn't do well, I would get real moody and feel insecure about everything. Also, I guess, deep down, I figured I was letting my dad down—disappointing him.

When I retired it got worse. I felt I was worthless without baseball—that I was a phony and that I was no good to myself or anyone else. It was at those times that I thought about death, and sometimes, like I said before, I wished it would come sooner than later.

Tom: When Billy Martin died in that car crash, how did you feel?

Mickey: I felt horrible. Billy and I used to joke about whose liver would give out first. We never thought about dying like he did. I felt alone and scared. I really missed Billy. Of course, my drinking eventually took care of my liver, just like Billy and me talked about.

Tom: What about what Chris was saying about male menopause—andropause?

Mickey: Sounds like a bunch of BS to me, but, hey, what do I know? I sure got moodier the older I got, and suffered some deep depression. I also got a lot fatter and my knees hurt more, too. But, I just called it, "getting older," and let it go at that. Nowadays guys have a lot more information. They should pay attention and do whatever they can to make life better for them and for people around them.

Maybe if I knew that what I was feeling was caused by hormone changes I would have gotten help earlier instead of hiding my fears in the bottle—maybe.

Tom: Would you have seen a counselor or a therapist?

Mickey: Maybe. Well, no, actually, probably not. I should have, but I would have been too bullheaded and embarrassed. No matter what I knew or what people would have told me, I think I probably still needed a crisis, like the one with Danny and Kaye when they checked into Betty Ford, before I would have asked for help. Stupid, but that's the truth. Like I tried to tell kids right before I died—don't be like me. I really screwed up.

Tom: Sounds like you still feel guilty?

Mickey: I guess that's the word—guilty. I know I shouldn't feel that way, but when I think about all the mistakes I made and the lives I messed with, it's hard not to feel guilty.

I really do believe that everyone who mattered to me forgave me before I died, but I was never able to get to the place where I could forgive myself. Like I said before, I was getting close, but I ran out of time. Of course, we always think we will have time to make up for things we did and said, but then, all of a sudden, the years are gone and so are we.

The Professor Speaks
About Men, Healthcare, and Personal Responsibility

Tom: Do men and women respond differently to healthcare and personal responsibility, Professor?

Professor Edwards: Yes, of course. Like in every other aspect of life, men and women handle health and responsibility in somewhat different ways.

Tom: For instance?

Professor Edwards: Let's take the case of the company CEO, as an example. This, by the way, is such a tragedy and one that could have easily been avoided.

Tom: You're talking about Harvey Martin's cancer.

Professor Edwards: Well, more about Harvey dying from this cancer, but yes. Harvey's reaction is pretty typical for men his age. Instead of getting regular annual checkups, he waited until the symptoms were so severe that he couldn't ignore them.

Guys, in general—all ages—don't want to talk about anything they think will make them look weak or vulnerable. We talked about this earlier, but it's the old Law of the Jungle mentality. Chris is right; Harvey may well die from embarrassment, failure to take responsibility for his health, and foolish, misguided pride.

Tom: And, women are different?

Professor Edwards: Women outlive men by seven years on average. Also, age-adjusted data indicates that the number of men who die from heart disease is double the number of women who die from heart disease and the incidence of stroke is 19 percent higher among men. Just as significant is the fact that 50 percent more men die of cancer than women, and men are at least 25 percent less likely than women to visit a doctor.

Certainly, a significant reason for the difference boils down to how men and women respond to the three key areas of personal health.

Tom: The three key areas of personal health?

Professor Edwards: Yes. They are:

• Medical Self-Responsibility

• Early Detection

• Early Intervention

When ill, you have a responsibility to seek help, ask questions, give complete and honest answers to questions asked of you, and, if time and circumstance warrant, to seek information and advice from as many other reliable resources as you can.

On the prevention side, it means that you have to pay attention to what's happening with your body, mind, and spirit—that you use your head when it comes to diet, exercise, alcohol consumption, stress, sense of purpose, and other factors that impact your physical, emotional, and spiritual health.

Certainly, there are underserved inner-city and rural populations where we need to do a better job with basic health education and affordable access to health services, but in general, people know what's good for them, what's not, and have reasonable access to healthcare.

When Harvey first saw blood, you can't tell me that he didn't get a little concerned. And, when it continued, he certainly knew that it was a bad sign— a sign that something was seriously wrong. And yet *still* he didn't tell anyone or go to the doctor.

Also, look at Lou, Ted, and Troy. They all know that their lifestyle choices are, at best, less than optimal. Even Chris must know that his obsession with exercise is unhealthy. But, other than make jokes and throw sarcastic barbs, nobody is taking any action. At some level, Tom, all these guys know that they are headed for trouble—they see it coming, but still they refuse to do anything about it.

There are two things that Mickey keeps coming back to—he makes it clear that he is fully responsible for what happened to him in life, and he regrets the fact that he ran out of time. Also, he doesn't plead ignorance. He doesn't say that he didn't know that what he was doing was harmful or unhealthy, he just said that he thought he would have time to change—later. He said the same things earlier when he was talking about the advice he would give the young Mickey Charles Mantle.

I guarantee you that at one time or another Lou has said to himself that he's going to lose weight, quit smoking, and cut back on all the fat and salt in his diet. Also, when Troy says that he is "young and free," he is really saying that when he's older he may change, but, for now, this is the kind of life he's going to lead. And, my guess is that, at some level, Ted thinks he is still "sowing wild oats" and that he will settle down, "someday."

Tom: You're saying that guys see the trouble coming but don't do anything about it?

Professor Edwards: That's exactly what I am saying. Tom, you were in the military, right? And, as I remember, you were stationed at a radar site in Alaska during Vietnam and the Cold War era?

Tom: Yes, that's right.

Professor Edwards: Okay, so let's think of this in terms of radar. What's the purpose of radar?

Tom: Well, the purpose for us at Indian Mountain Air Force Station was to monitor U.S. air space so that we could detect inbound Russian aircraft or missiles as early as possible and send a warning to the command center at Elmendorf Air Force Base in Anchorage. If they determined the threat was real, they scrambled fighter jets to fly out to take a closer look and, if need be, neutralize the threat.

Professor Edwards: As a radar operator, what would happen if you saw inbound objects on your radar scope but did nothing about it?

Tom: Well, besides getting court-martialed and possibly thrown in the brink, if the threat was real, we might get shot at, bombed, and maybe killed. Or, if not us, someone else that we were supposed to be protecting.

Professor Edwards: Okay, so let's use radar as a metaphor for men and life. Often we have "blips" or warning signs that pop up on our radar screens. These blips deal with things like health, children, intimate relationships, or work. We may not understand exactly what they are, but we know they exist. Now, if it was actual radar, my guess is that the radar operator would take a closer look to determine if the blip was moving, or if it was something stationary like a mountain or maybe a false echo caused by something like sunspots. If the blip was moving, the operator would then try to determine how fast it was approaching, how high it was flying, and whether or not it was friend or foe. Right?

Tom: Sounds like you've been there, Professor. That's about it. And, if it was not immediately determined that the blip was friendly, the radar operator would notify his supervisor who would put in motion a series of procedures to definitively identify the object and remove the threat.

Professor Edwards: So, the operator would never say that he was too busy to check out the blip, assume that it was a false echo, or trust that if he let it go through, someone else would pick it up and neutralize the threat?

Tom: I get your point. You're saying that men often ignore threats or assume that they aren't real and that, even if they are, someone else will take care of them. Is that about it?

Professor Edwards: Bingo! Not only do we ignore and assume, we are outraged and feel victimized when we look up and our personal sky is filled with problems, the bombs are falling, and shrapnel is whizzing by our heads.

This is when we say stupid things like, "I didn't see that coming," "I was blind-sided," "It just appeared out of the blue," and other classic denials. Then, to make matters worse, we whine as we point fingers at the government, kids, bosses, wives, parents, girlfriends, or even the weather.

As I have said before, until we live a life accented by self-responsibility, early detection, and early intervention, we will forever be helpless victims blaming others for our poor health, personal failures, and missed career opportunities.

.chapter
nine

Oh, you, Kid…
Men and Kids

"A child needs your love most when he deserves it least."
— Erma Bombeck

It was a fairly easy week. Betty Jacobson, our executive vice president, is now the acting president and pretty much a shoe-in to replace Harvey. She's been with the company for over twenty years and is well qualified. Pleasant, but not what you would call friendly. Betty's a stickler for discipline and has little tolerance for excuses. Much of the week has been spent in meetings. Betty and I will work fine together and I'm glad she'll be in charge.

I did manage to play ball last night and had a great time. Ben came out to watch the old man chug around the bases. I hit two doubles! I don't know who was happier, Ben or me.

Good thing I still have Ben because the girls, in particular Erica, my fifteen-year-old, are giving Dad the cold shoulder. No matter what I do, I seem to anger or embarrass them. Katy, thirteen, still sneaks hugs, but as far as Erica is concerned, I'm "like totally poison." My only consolation is that she's that way with Laurie, too. The difference is that where Laurie fights with her constantly, I just walk away or hold it until I burst, and then feel guilty and want to buy her things.

Talk at the lunch table is all about kids. Jim finally spoke up at the begin-
ning of the week and told us about his sixteen-year-old daughter, Shelley.
Seems Shelley's been involved with drugs since the eighth grade. She got busted
selling marijuana and the court ordered her into rehab or juvenile detention,
her choice. That's why Jim's been missing so much work. Like a lot of fathers,
he doesn't have a clue how to talk with his kids. His marriage is also suffering
because of it. On top of everything, his mother-in-law has emphysema to the
point where she needs to be placed in a nursing home. He's taking it really hard
and is just about at the end of his rope. Jerry Spatalie's suicide didn't help his
current, dismal outlook on life. At today's lunch, we continue talking about
kids, dads, and how to bring the two together. At the end of lunch, two women
from the plant join us.

Harvey continues to slip fast. Death could just be a matter of days.
Although concerned, none of the guys—except Lou and I—were that close to
the boss and feel that a visit would be an intrusion. Given Harvey's current
state, they're right. Lou went to see him at his home and has been pretty shook
up ever since. However, as always with Lou, he eventually dodges life's
awkward moments with humor.

"Any change?"

Lou asks the same question each time he sees me. "No, Lou. No change."

"I know Harvey has a couple of sons," says Jim, "How many grandkids?"

Picturing his office filled with crayon stick figures, rainbows, and photos, I
reply, "Six. And they all have Grandpa wrapped around their little fingers." I
smile, thinking of Rory, the baby. "The oldest, Maureen, is twelve."

"Yeah," says Lou, "you should see Harvey with those kids. I've never seen
a grownup get along as well with kids as Harvey does. They run to him whenever
they see the old man. He eats it up! Spoils 'em, rotten!"

Jim looks up, "That's because they're not his. They don't live in his house.
I bet it wasn't that way with his own kids. Didn't one of them get arrested for
shoplifting when he was a teenager? It was in the paper, as I remember."

"Greg. Yeah, stupid kid stuff," says Lou. "A CD or something like that. But,
because his old man was a hot shot and on the outs with the publisher over some
advertising contract, the paper ran with it. Any other kid and they would have left
it alone," he adds with a glare. "It's like President Bush's kids and the time they
got busted for beer.

"Having watched those kids grow up," Lou adds, "I can tell you they've always been a tight-knit family. Harvey loves this place, but Jane and the kids always came first—always."

"I'm just telling you, Lou," says Jim, lifting his eyebrows, raising his voice, and tapping his fork against his plate, "It's not that goddamn easy. You give them everything and they break your heart and drive you crazy. When they're little, it's one thing, but when they become teenagers, it's totally different. MTV, drugs, booze, boys. Christ, the next thing I expect is for one or *both* of them to get pregnant.

"If that happens, I'm telling ya, they're out, goddamn it! I got enough problems without more kids running around the place. Either they're out, or I'm out!"

Everybody is a bit stunned by Jim's outburst and hesitant to say anything. Everybody, of course, but Chris.

"Whoa, where did that come from? I thought we were talking about Harvey's kids! Listen to yourself, Jim. Keep talking like that, and that's exactly what will happen," he says with authority.

"Christ, Iverson, I'm so sick of your sanctimonious know-it-all bullshit. What the *hell* do you know about it? Huh? What the hell do you know?"

Characteristically unfazed by criticism, Chris responds, "I'm just telling you that if you keep predicting that your kids are going to screw up, you're going help make it happen. In some way, Shelley's probably trying to get back at you for the way you treat her."

"All right, smart guy, you take her, take 'em both. In fact, take my wife and her pain-in-the-ass-mother too—you can have 'em all. I quit!" And, with this last outburst, Jim gets up and leaves the table.

"What?…What?" Chris asks as the rest of us stare at him. "What did I do?"

"Chris," I say as tactfully as I can, "sometimes, you come off a little strong. Jim's obviously having a real tough time right now. He doesn't need you telling him he screwed up."

"Well, he did screw up," says Chris undeterred, "and, if he doesn't watch it, he'll get those grandkids he's so afraid of. Screwed-up parents make screwed-up kids. Period."

"It must be wonderful," Ted says, "having all the answers, Chris. I hope your baby grows up perfect, my friend. Of course, if she doesn't, my guess is that it will be your wife's fault. Right?"

No comment from Chris.

Lou—who can't stand the tension any longer—says, "Okay, okay, one day, a little girl looks at her mother's hair and asks, sadly, 'Mommy, why is some of your hair white?' The mother replies, 'Well, every time you do something wrong and make me cry or unhappy, one of my hairs turns white.' The little girl thinks for a minute, and then says, 'Mommy, *all* of Grandma's hairs are white!'"

"Hey, Lou," shoots Troy speaking for the first time today, "I saw your mama and she's bald—what's up with that?"

Lou hurls a grape across the table. Troy ducks and the grape hits Gloria from accounting in the back of the head.

"My God," shouts the tall red-head. "You would think you guys were still in middle school," she adds with a mixture of amusement and annoyance. "Keep it up and I'll call over the assistant principal and he'll paddle the lot of you."

"Gloria," asks Ted, "I've got a question for you. Who's primarily responsible for raising the kids? The mom or the dad?"

"Both," she says without hesitation. "Unless there's a divorce, then it's the mother's day-to-day responsibility."

"Why should the mother get the kids?" asks Troy.

"Because, women make better parents."

"What? How can you say that?" asks Ted. "My kids adore me."

"That's got nothing to do with being a good parent," Gloria shoots back. "Playing catch, goofing-off, and going to the movies—that's the easy stuff. Try getting them to do their homework, dealing out the discipline, mending a broken heart, shopping, listening to their problems, washing their clothes, cooking their food, cleaning the house, and going to school functions. Being a good parent doesn't mean picking out the fun stuff and leaving the tough part to someone else."

Barb from sales jumps in, "On top of that, throw in a sixty-hour work-week plus trying to look nice for creeps like you!"

Obviously, we've touched a nerve.

"Gloria, come here for a moment, will you?" I say. "Bring your coffee. You, too, Barb."

Having finished their meals, the two forty-something women join our table.

"Help us out here," I plead. "You've got kids in high school; how do you talk to teenagers? Jim can't seem to get through to his girls, Erica has just decided that I'm invisible, and Katy's not far behind—I can't talk to them anymore. Help!"

"First of all," begins Gloria, "have you tried *listening* instead of talking? Men are all alike. You think everything can be solved in the time it takes to drink a beer, watch a ball game, or…." She pauses and thinks better about saying what she was thinking, holds back for a second, and then continues, "Kids need someone to just listen to them—no judgment, no lecture, no stories about 'when I was your age…,' none of that. Just full, undivided attention—on them. Their needs—the kids' needs—not yours."

Barb picks up the lead, "Men always want to fix things. They somehow get off on being the big shot with all the answers." All our eyes go to Chris, as Barb continues, "And, if they can't fix it, they take it personally, or totally blame someone else for the mess and then just walk away."

"Wait, wait," says Ted, "not all men. Just Chris, here, just Chris. Some of us are perfect. Ain't that right, Troy?"

"There's another thing," adds Gloria leaning across the table and pointing her finger at Ted. "Why is everything a joke with you guys? Being charming is one thing, but a laugh, a wink, and a nudge are not always the solutions. Sometimes, you actually have to understand a situation before you shoot off your mouth! I heard you talking to Jim, Chris, and no wonder he left the table. Jim's problems are no secret around here—you guys talk plenty loud enough," she adds with a frown.

"It's obvious that he's going crazy trying to *solve* his wife's menopause, *solve* his mother-in-law's illness, and *solve* his kid's growing-up. These are not 'problems' to solve! They are life events that need attention, compassion, understanding, and a sympathetic ear! And, instead of just listening to Jim's concerns, you, Chris, tried to fix him! We heard you! Quit trying to fix everything!!!"

Realizing she's getting too wound-up, Gloria takes a deep breath, smiles, and says, "Sorry, but I have this conversation with my husband, Terry, all the time. It seems to stick for awhile and then he slips back into playing Mr. Fix-It."

Not really knowing what to say, we just sit and stare at each other.

"And, guys," adds Barb, "your daughters, in particular, really need your understanding and support. You are the models for the future men in their life. How you treat them impacts their self-esteem and confidence. Talk with them, play with them, take them places where you go. Make them feel special. Same goes for boys, but even more so for your girls."

Wow! Way too much for Lou.

"Hey, wait a minute. Not all men try to fix things. This man and woman got up for work one morning," says Lou, nervously taking a bite of his second piece of pie, "and the woman says, 'Honey, the refrigerator needs fixing.' The man says, 'Do I look like the Maytag repair man?' Then she says, 'The car also needs fixing.' 'Do I look like Mr. Goodwrench?' So, the man goes on to work, and when he finally gets home, the woman says, 'Oh, I got the car and the refrigerator fixed. The man next door fixed them.' The husband asks, 'Well, how much did he charge?' She says, 'He said I can either sleep with him or bake him a cake.' The husband asks, 'What kind of cake did you bake?' 'Do I look like Betty Crocker?' she replies."

Troy and Ted laugh, Chris and I shake our heads, and Gloria and Barb leave the table.

What Would Mickey Say?
About Men and Kids

Tom: What did being a father mean to you, Mick?

Mickey: I was twenty when Merlyn and I got married. I was just a kid myself when Mickey, Jr. was born in 1953. David was born two years later and then Billy in '58 and Danny in '60. So, there I was, twenty-eight years old with four kids. Like I said, I was just a kid, myself. I didn't know what to do when they were little. I left all the raising stuff to Merlyn. You know, school, chores, discipline—stuff like that. No excuse, but where I grew up, the kids were mom's. And, yes, I knew better, but I just didn't do anything about it. I still feel bad.

Tom: How did your boys feel about it?

Mickey: They always said I was too hard on myself and that it wasn't that bad. But, like I said, I know better. It *was* that bad. I can't help but think if I had been around and been more attentive, Billy might still be alive and the rest of them would not have needed rehab. The boys needed a dad, and I wasn't there for any of them.

Tom: Not to let you off the hook, Mick, but the nature of your job kept you on the road. There are a lot of dads who don't get to spend time with their kids. They feel bad, but they don't beat themselves up about it, and their kids turn out fine.

Mickey: Listen, I appreciate what you're saying, Tom, but it wasn't just that. It was true that I found out about Mickey, Jr. from the public address announcer during a game in Cleveland, and that Danny was born when I was in Spring Training. I guess that was unavoidable, given my job. But, as an example of how I let Merlyn and the kids down, I was out screwing around with Billy Martin when little Billy was born. I knew she was close to delivering, but I chose to hang out and get drunk with Billy instead of be by her side. And, like I mentioned before, there was the time I shoved Merlyn around just two days before David was born.

Merlyn used to joke that the kids enjoyed the glimpses they got of me four months out of every year. I gave them lots of money and things, but no discipline and no direction and—maybe worst of all—no time. At least not until they were old enough to take to the bar.

Tom: Did you at least go to their games, their school events, and things like that?

Mickey: No, not really. I used to beg off saying that I didn't want to mess up things by attracting a crowd, but the truth is that was really just an excuse. I probably wouldn't have gone anyway. I told you, Tom, I was not a good dad. I just never learned. Maybe some guys come by it naturally, but not me. Hell, I kept thinking about my dad and wishing he were still around to guide me, so why would I think I had what it takes to guide someone else's life? Most of the time, we had it reversed—the boys took care of me. I was the kid and they were the parents. Pretty sad, huh? Pretty sad.

The Professor Speaks
About Men and Kids

Tom: Sounds like a classic male/female, nature/nurture question, Professor. So, is Gloria right, are women naturally better parents than men? Or is it like Mickey implied, that parenting is a skill that's taught, and he just never learned how?

Professor Edwards: I think you're really asking two questions. One: If the kids turn out okay, is it because of their gene pool or because of the way they're raised? Two: If only one parent can raise a child, who would do a better job, the father or the mother?

Tom: That's what I'm asking, yes.

Professor Edwards: Judith Harris did a pretty thorough job on question number one in her book, *The Nurture Assumption*, which claims that the main influence on the nurturing side of children's development is not parents, but the peer group. In other words, while nature (in the form of genetic characteristics) certainly influences intelligence and personality characteristics, the specific contribution of parents to the nurturing process is, in many cases, less influential than the impact of the peer group.

Tom: Okay, so you're saying that the latest evidence suggests that environment plays a stronger role than heredity. But, that still doesn't answer my question about parenting. Who does a better job—a man or a woman?

Professor Edwards: Gender isn't the question. There is no solid evidence that supports a purely genetic argument for either sex. The issue isn't *who* is raising the kids, but *how* they are raising them and *what* and *who* are the other influencers. We can't argue with the fact that negligent or abusive parents (moms and dads) have a devastating effect on children's perceptions of the world, and hence influence their entire thinking processes and actions. At the same time, Harris's research reminds us just how important peer influence really is, and this means that both men and women play a critical role. Children need as many responsible adults as possible to pay attention to where they are going, who they are going with, and what they are doing. Wise parents not only develop strong parenting skills and participate positively in their children's lives, they also continuously scan the others who interact with their children on a regular basis. When they anticipate problems, they intervene, guiding their children away from negative influences. Parents and guardians can't block all the harmful television, radio, movies, and schoolyard influences; however, they can guide them toward more positive influences through involvement in activities and with different peer groups.

Tom: So Mickey was right. He was a bad parent who didn't know how to be a good father. He should have taken a more active role in guiding his kids.

Professor Edwards: Close. I think he would be the first person to tell you that he knew better—if in fact, he says that he did. So, the argument that he didn't know how is weak, at best. Even though he was reflecting the norm of the day, one that placed Mom in the home and Dad at work, he knew that he could have and should have been more involved.

The sad part, of course, is that not only could it have had a positive impact on the way the kids were raised, he also missed the pure joy that comes from spending time with your kids. This is the part that I think really bothered him—all the missed moments.

Tom: Is there a formula for being a good dad? Or a good mom, for that matter?

Professor Edwards: Sure. And it's pretty basic. Give your kids time, attention, love, affection, and guidance. Oh, and never underestimate the power of being a role model. I just mentioned that peers and outside forces have a huge impact upon early development, but kids will look to key adults for lessons on how to behave as an adult. Abusive parents are more likely to produce the next generation of abusers. Parents who live a life accented by tobacco, poor nutrition, and little physical exercise are more likely to create a new generation of unhealthy adults. Bigots tend to beget bigots, and so on. Hypocritical lectures and stupid expressions like, "Do as I say and not as I do," ring hollow with kids and bring to mind another phrase: "Your actions are so loud, I can't hear what you are saying!"

Tom, keep in mind that the opposite is also true. A kind neighbor, a trusting teacher, a helpful stranger—all have a positive impact. It may sound corny, but Hillary Clinton was right, it does take a village to raise healthy, happy, and productive children.

chapter
ten

D-i-v-o-r-c-e
Promises Made, Promises Broken...

On Monday, after his routine stop at Travis Pointe Country Club for a couple drinks with the boys, Ted went home to an empty house. I mean empty. While he was at work pinching the ladies and telling sexist jokes, Lucy took the two little girls and all the furniture and left town. She left him his clothes, a letter found in his suit pocket, the food in the refrigerator, and a note...

Ted,

I have had enough. I can't take it anymore and I won't let you do this to our girls. I've tried and tried and tried, but no more...

The ongoing pain and humiliation are more than I can bear. In fact, I won't bear it any longer!!!

You can probably guess where we have gone, but do not, I repeat, <u>do not</u> follow us. My lawyer will contact you in a few days.

Tell "Love Ya Lilly" she can have you (yes, as you see, I found her sleazy and disgusting letter— Christ, I hope she screws better than she spells...). By the way, does Lilly know about Jill, Veronica, Sue, and God only knows how many other tramps you have waiting for you in some honky-tonk bar?

PS. I hope you rot in hell!

How do I know this is what the note said? Because Ted showed it to me right after he was served papers on Tuesday morning. He wanted to use his accumulated sick days to head to Texas and chase down Lucy and the girls. Lucy's folks live in Austin and Ted is certain that's where she and the kids have gone. I told him to take it easy and just calm down before he did anything. After a few minutes, he broke down and sobbed like a baby. He kept saying how he couldn't believe that she would do this to him—that she would intentionally hurt him. How could she just take the kids and go? He still doesn't get it.

So, he's gone. I gave him the time off. However, when he comes back, he has another surprise. Betty Jacobson sent a memo out on Wednesday outlining a very clear zero-tolerance sexual harassment policy. She encouraged any woman who has been harassed to come forward with names. Guess whose name is at the top of the list?

Harvey passed away Tuesday. His service was held on Thursday. We forfeited our game Thursday night.

Today's talk centers around dating, marriage, and divorce. Jim continues to dip into his bank of sick days and was again a no-show both for last night's game and today's lunch.

Sounding lost, the Big Guy says, "Things like yesterday [Harvey's funeral] make ya think. And, I don't wanna think. Too depressing. Very sad."

"When you add in Ted's wife taking off with the kids," adds Troy, "it makes for one hell of a week.

"I told him this would happen—didn't I?" Troy asks no one in particular. "Stupid jerk."

"Actually, Troy," I say, "I believe your words were something like, 'A little extra-curricular activity is good for a relationship' and, 'What Mama doesn't know can't hurt her.' "

"Yeah, well, his problem is that he got caught," says Troy, oblivious to the point. "Nobody would have gotten hurt if he hadn't kept that stupid note."

"Ya see," mumbles Lou through his cheeseburger, "that's why I never got married. Everybody cheats on everybody else. I'd go nuts if that happened. Friggin' nuts!"

"You don't cheat if you love the person," says Chris, sitting down at the table. "You just don't. No matter how tempted you are."

"Ain't got nothin' to do with love, Christopher," adds Troy. "It's all in the genes. Men are not meant to be with one woman." Waving his right arm over the cafeteria, he continues, "Men are meant to spread their seed everywhere they can."

"Why don't you ask Ted how he feels about your little theory?" I ask. "My hunch is that he's changed his tune."

"For an old guy, Tom, you're pretty naïve," says Chris. "My guess is that Ted feels pretty much the same way Lover Boy, here, feels." He points at Troy. "He's just pissed and scared because he got caught. If she takes him back—and my money says she will—he'll do it again."

"No argument, here," says Troy.

"Look at all the U.S. presidents who screwed around," says Lou. "I don't mean just Kennedy and Clinton," he continues, "I bet they all did. Hell, I bet old Georgie Porgie was gettin' it on while Martha was home baking him a cherry pie."

"Like I said," perks up Troy, "it's in the genes. Guys can't help it. We're made that way!"

"All right, one more Clinton joke," says Lou bouncing up and down in his chair and rubbing his hands together. "A new ABC poll asked 1,000 women if they would have sex with Clinton. 70 percent said, 'Never again.'"

"You guys don't want to hear this," says Chris, "but one of the most beautiful relationships in recorded history was between a U.S. president and his wife. John Adams, our second president, and his wife, Abigail."

"You got that right, Lycra Boy," Lou says as he winks at Troy, "we don't want to hear that fluffy chick stuff."

"You know who I feel sorry for?" asks Troy. "The kids. Good thing they're young," he says, shaking his head and changing his tune. "I went through this when I was a teenager, and it was hell. Everyone knew what was going on except Mom. I tried to tell her, but she didn't want to hear it. My sister's still screwed up because of it. Married three times, and each one worse than the one before."

With a smirk, Chris lifts his head, "She's probably screwed up because of man's uncontrollable need to spread his seed, right, Troy?"

"Okay," says Lou, "more information than I need to know. Here's one I *know* you haven't heard," he rushes to say before Troy gives out any more family secrets. "A guy sticks his head into a barber shop and asks, 'How long before I can get a haircut?' The barber looks around the shop and says, 'About two hours.' The guy leaves.

"A few days later the same guy sticks his head in the door and asks, 'How long before I can get a haircut?' The barber looks around at his shop full of customers and says, 'About two hours.' The guy leaves.

"A week later the same guy sticks his head in the shop and asks, 'How long before I can get a haircut?' The barber looks around the shop and says 'About an hour-and-a-half.' The guy leaves.

"The barber looks over at a friend in the shop and says 'Hey, Bill, follow that guy and see where he goes.' In a little while, Bill comes back into the shop laughing hysterically. The barber asks, 'Bill, where did he go when he left here?'

"Bill looks up and says, 'To your house.'"

What Would Mickey Say?
About Marriage and Divorce

Tom: Mick, you openly admit to being a bad husband. What would you have done differently?

Mickey: During our marriage I wasn't much of a husband, that's true, but Merlyn and I never stopped loving each other. Throughout our forty-three years, I never wanted a divorce, and I never wanted any other woman to have my name. That was Merlyn's as long as she wanted it.

Tom: But what went wrong?

Mickey: Hell, I don't know, but keep in mind that I was only twenty years old when we got married. Heck, I didn't want to get married. I loved Merlyn, sure, but I didn't want to get married.

Tom: Then, why did you?

Mickey: I guess, in part, because I knew how much it meant to my dad. He was pretty sick at the time and I knew that it would make him happy to see us married. My age sure didn't matter to him. He was only seventeen when he married my mom.

Merlyn used to say that my dad was the second happiest person at the wedding after her, and that I was somewhere in the top five. I guess she was right. She was also right when she said that, in my view, marriage was a party with special added attractions. You see, when I was twenty, the party had lots of pretty girls and plenty of free booze. It was just getting started and I didn't want marriage to mess it up. A stupid notion, I know, but I'm just being honest.

Tom: How did Merlyn react to your notion of marriage?

Mickey: Oh, over the years, I think she knew it was kind of a sick relationship, but even when I came home with lipstick on my collar and smelling of perfume, her philosophy was that what happened on the road was outside of what happened at home, so it didn't really matter. The idea of one-night stands was tolerable, as long as it didn't turn into a full-blown affair.

Tom: What finally happened that caused you to leave for good in 1988?

Mickey: I never really left for good—not really. We spent holidays, birthdays, and other special occasions together. It's just that we couldn't live under the same roof anymore. My behavior with other women was so out of control that I got tired of hiding it and telling lies. It was easier to just leave.

Tom: How did Merlyn take your leaving?

Mickey: She wasn't too pleased, that's for sure. There was a lot of yelling and throwing things at the beginning, but she settled down. I told her she could have a divorce if she wanted, but I sure didn't. I just didn't want to live with her and have to give up other women. She told me she couldn't imagine not being Mrs. Mickey Mantle, so we eventually settled into being each other's best friend and actually got along better by not living together. Like I said, she figured it was a pretty sick elationship, but it seemed to work for us. Shoot, long before I left, she used to tell people that we were married...but only in a small geographical area of my mind.

Tom: I can't imagine that money was a problem for her, but who took care of her emotional needs?

Mickey: Because my drinking got worse after I left, I had to leave that up to the boys. I figured I just couldn't take care of her or the boys. This was another big guilt trip for me. I felt so bad, but I just didn't know what to do.

Tom: No offensive, Mick, but isn't that just another cop out, or pure denial? Like with the boys, you probably knew what to do, you just chose not to do it. Don't tell me you blamed the booze?

Mickey: Oh, yeah, sure. I blamed the booze, I blamed Merlyn, I blamed my dad, I blamed everyone but me. It wasn't until later that I realized how much time I spent in denial. We both did—both Merlyn and me. I guess that goes for the boys, too.

I guess in today's world, Merlyn would be called an enabler or a codependent. Even when she knew I was screwing around, she used to treat me like a king. Most of the time we would pretend that we had the best marriage around. I remember on our nineteenth wedding anniversary I sent her a note saying that I hoped the next nineteen were as happy as the first nineteen. Our response to trouble was to do our best to ignore it, and pretend everything was just fine.

Tom: Back to my original question, Mick. What would you have done differently?

Mickey: I'm no expert on giving advice, but I sure would have waited to get married. I was just a kid from the farm and hadn't really experienced a whole lot before me and Merlyn got married. I suppose both Merlyn and my dad figured that if we didn't get married soon, I might find someone else. In my dad's case, he liked Merlyn and felt she was "my kind." Merlyn just wanted to get married. I'm not saying she didn't love me—she did—no question about it. It's just that she probably liked the idea of marriage almost as much.

So, my advice would be to wait until you've done some living; don't marry just because it will make someone else happy. And, when you do marry, make sure you are committed to staying with that person—forever. Oh yeah, and whatever you do, don't think you can change someone once you're married. What you see is what you get. Men seem to understand that better than women. They seem to think, "Oh, he'll change once we're married." I'm telling you, it doesn't work that way.

Tom: Good advice—anything else?

Mickey: Yeah. Don't pretend everything is okay when it isn't. We could have solved many problems early on if we were honest with one another. I was too damn stubborn, and I suppose Merlyn was too proud or maybe too scared to call me on certain things. One more thing—get professional help from someone like a marriage counselor if you can't seem to work things out on your own. Or, talk to your minister, rabbi, or your priest. Or, a good buddy. Funny, I could talk to Billy and Whitey about almost anything, but I never talked about my marriage or even about the kids, except to brag when they did something good.

My time at Betty Ford taught me the value of getting help when you need it—about getting things off your chest—about not being afraid to tell someone when you're feeling afraid. Man, I'm grateful for the eighteen months of sobriety I had afterwards, but I can't help think about all those friggin' years I wasted. Also, I can't help but think that if Merlyn and I had counseling in the early years, we may have been able to turn things around and build a good life for all of us. But, as I've said so many times, I was too soon old and too late smart.

The Professor Speaks
About Marriage and Divorce

Tom: Well, Professor?

Professor Edwards: No surprise Tom. A number of studies show that, on average, men, women, and children are happier living as a family unit. However, those averages conceal wide variations. Not all marriages are good, and neither are all single-family situations bad. Given Mickey's clear desire to live life as a single man, an argument could be made that early divorce may have been a wise consideration. Given the fact that no one disputes where Mick was on the "happy-at-the-wedding" scale, an early separation, intense counseling, and possibly a divorce may have avoided a tremendous amount of stress and turmoil for all the Mantles.

It's interesting to note that the studies suggest that Mickey is the one who would have suffered most if they had indeed gotten an early divorce. Married men enjoy better health and longevity and fewer psychological and behavioral problems than single men. Merlyn, on the other hand, may have faired better with a divorce. Women thrive in a stable, predictable marriage, but are likely to experience depression and numerous physical health problems when the marriage is shaky, as was the Mantle's. Merlyn's alcoholism, heart disease, and depression were certainly linked to a dysfunctional marriage. My guess is that, although the separation was difficult at first, there was a certain amount of peace that came when Mickey moved out—not at first, perhaps, but fairly quickly thereafter.

Tom: What makes for a risky marriage? Are there flags that signal danger ahead?

Professor Edwards: Marriages can be flagged according to risk ranging from those with a high likelihood of divorce to those with minimal risks. While certainly no ironclad guide, here's a look at the various types of marriages in descending order of risk.

1) *"I don't want to talk about it."*—*"Neither do I."* Pure denial. Both individuals live in a world of make-believe—a world where discomfort equates with failure, where discovery beckons only disaster. Best not talk about it for fear it is—or will become—real.
   Prognosis: Don't bother to freeze the wedding cake. Nobody will be around for the thaw.

2) *"Let's talk."*—*"I don't want to."* Usually with this couple, it is the wife who wants to talk and confront problems head-on, while the husband goes to great lengths not to share—or even admit—that he has feelings. Of course, in same-sex relationships, there is no gender distinction, but the roles exist just the same. One wants to talk until the wee hours of the night, and the other wants only to sleep and/or pretend that all is well.

Prognosis: If not you, keep in mind that there are always others who will be willing to listen, and then some. Don't say you didn't see it coming. Sure you did...you just didn't want to talk about it.

3) *"You're nice, but who are you, anyway?"* In this relationship, there are few common interests, activities, or friends. There is no passion—either positive or negative. They merely coexist without real conflict, affection, or sexual satisfaction.

   Prognosis: You may stay together but only due to inertia. Relationships and emotions at rest, tend to stay at rest. ZZZZZZZZZ*zzzzzzzzzzzzzzz*.

4) *"I hate you...I love you...I hate you...I love you!"* Fights worthy of a Hollywood epic followed by make-up sex that shakes the rafters. Eventually, however, the intensity becomes almost unbearable on both ends of the spectrum.

   Prognosis: Without long timeouts, one or both will collapse. Better than a relationship without any emotion, but still very shaky, and potentially dangerous when the make-up sex settles down to a subtle quiver. Watch out for Othello's Green-Eyed Monster...absent diligent safeguards, jealously will bite hard and gobble up both parties.

5) *"One + One = Three."* A relationship accented by warmth, consideration, and a sincere desire to help the other advance as an individual, including pursuing independent goals and, at times, independent friendships. Requires a deep level of trust and a strong sense of self-worth.

   Prognosis: Absolute Nirvana, If BOTH parties are secure, honest, open, willing to compromise, and highly sensitive to one another's needs. A rare relationship, but worth the initial effort it takes to build and maintain.

6) *"Me Tarzan, you Jane—and we both like it that way."* What we have come to think of as a "traditional" relationship where one person— usually the man, in heterosexual relationships— is the primary bread winner and the other partner takes on the majority of the nurturing and domestic responsibilities. These relationships work very well as long as each person continues to buy into the traditional role assignments.

   Prognosis: Best shot at celebrating that Golden Anniversary surrounded by all the grandchildren and great-grandchildren. Roles are clearly defined with minimal crossover. Easy to keep score and predict the outcome. Kind of like coloring within the lines. Nice and tidy. Not everyone's cup of tea, but statically, the clearest path to a long, happy, and fulfilling relationship.

It is interesting to note that women are most psychologically and physically sensitive to the various types of relationships. Women in the first three types of relationships described above suffer the most emotional and physical health problems. Significantly fewer troubles occur for women in volatile relationships, and little physical or psychological distress is in store for women in mutually supportive and traditional relationships.

Men have a difficult time with the first two, but suffer only negligible impact from the other types of relationships.

Of course, it doesn't take a seven-figure study to show us that, overall, marriages and relationships accented by contempt, belligerence, denial, and withdrawal are doomed, while those characterized by respect, trust, support, and value tend to flourish.

Tom: So what happens when two people get divorced? Who suffers more, men or women?

Professor Edwards: Well, actually, at the beginning—particularly when children are involved—divorce is horrible for everyone. Starting with the first served papers, anger, guilt, confusion, resentment, bitterness, and fear dominate. "Why?" "How could you?" "What if...?" "What now?" are common exclamations that accompany divorce. However, studies show that beginning in year two, there is a gradual recovery, and by the sixth year, data indicates that, for the most part, both parties have moved on with their lives.

Women tend to move faster than men, but both men and women emerge with healthier perspectives on life leading to new relationships, hobbies, and opportunities. About 70 percent of men and 60 percent of women remarry, with the remainder seeking intimacy without marriage through dating, cohabitating, and deep, meaningful relationships with family and friends.

Tom: What about the kids?

Professor Edwards: While most adults recover whole from divorce, the general consensus is that children do not fair as well—at least not initially. Both young children and adolescents in divorced and remarried families have been found to have, on average, more social, emotional, academic, and behavioral problems than kids in two-parent, non-divorced families.

E. Mavis Hetherington, author of *For Better or For Worse: Divorce Reconsidered*, found twice as many serious psychological disorders and behavioral problems—such as teenage pregnancy, dropping out of school, substance abuse, unemployment, and marital breakups—among the offspring of divorced parents as compared to the children of non-divorced families. Sadly, she notes, this is a closer association than between smoking and cancer.

Fortunately, however, according to Ms. Hetherington, the troubled youngsters remain a relatively small proportion of the total. In her study, she found that 75 percent to 80 percent of children and adolescents from divorced families, after a period of initial disruption, are able to cope with the divorce and their new life situation and develop into reasonably or exceptionally well-adjusted individuals.

Keep in mind, Tom, that many of the adjustment problems in parents and children—and much of the inept parenting and destructive family relations, which policy makers have attributed to divorce— are actually present before divorce. Being in a dysfunctional family has taken its toll long before the breakup occurs. I don't believe that either Mickey or Merlyn would disagree that there were serious problems in the family long before Mickey decided to leave.

Again, according to Ms. Hetherington and other researchers, it comes as no surprise that several studies show that adults and children who are mature, stable, self-regulated, and adaptable are more likely able to cope with the challenges of divorce. Those who are neurotic, antisocial, and impulsive—and who lack a sense of their own efficacy—are likely to have these characteristics exacerbated by the breakup. In other words, the psychologically poor get poorer after a divorce, while the rich often get richer.

chapter
eleven

Hello, Betty...Goodbye, Ted!
Leadership and Men at Work

*A*s expected, the board of directors moved quickly and offered Betty Jacobson the position of president and CEO of Erie Ball Bearings. I've worked with Betty for years and couldn't be more pleased. She'll do a great job.

One of her first executive tasks was to ask Ted for his resignation.

Ted leaving came as no big surprise. Once Jane Myers from the cafeteria staff came forward with tales of fanny pinching, propositions, and lewd jokes, a line quickly formed outside of Betty's door. The game of "Oh yeah? I can top that..." played on for much of Betty's first days at the helm.

The "fumigation" (as Gloria referred to it) occurred with such efficiency that Ted never saw what hit him. Spewing barbs at every woman he'd ever known, he was gone before lunch. Calls to key clients and replacement interviews are already scheduled for this afternoon.

Actually, Betty gave Ted a break. She could have easily fired him. However, to avoid further embarrassment to Lucy, and to minimize disruption around the shop, Betty let him walk out the door instead of ordering a security escort. While some of the women wanted to see him publicly humiliated, most were simply glad he was leaving. As for me, I had no idea Ted had caused so much disruption and personal distress. Obviously, this does not speak well for my performance as head of HR. I never saw the adverse impact his behavior was having on the staff;

I was just angry because he was deceiving his family. All told, I was feeling more than just a little guilty that I didn't speak up more than I did. Of course, if it was my fanny he was pinching, I probably would have felt very different and certainly would have done something about it.

After initial reactions to the surprise dismissal (the men were surprised—not the women), the lunch table talk settles into a discussion of corporate re-organization, management styles, men working for women, and the importance of work-life balance.

Also, earlier in the day, Jim found out that he was passed over for department head—again. No one, including Jim, is surprised. However, true to form, no one talks about it.

Mickey talks about working for various managers. He also talks about his short-lived coaching job with the Yankees. As for work-life balance, the disproportionate time spent with baseball-related activities (on and off the field) left guilt that haunted him until the day he died.

Professor Edwards talks about leadership.

"Wrong place, wrong time," says Troy as he sits down with his tray.

"What are you talking about?" asks Lou, pulling up with the usual trio of burgers dripping with ketchup.

"Ted," continues Troy, "he got canned because we got a skirt running the show. She's probably pissed at her old man and decided to take it out on Ted. Hell, maybe she's a dyke."

Amazed that even someone as brash and, at times, as stupid as Troy would spew such homophobic and sexist garbage, I open my mouth to speak, but as usual, Chris beats me to it.

"He got canned because he's a moron!" shouts Chris, an artery thumping in his neck. "A moron who got exactly what was coming to him. And Troy," Chris says in more measured tones, "what's with you, anyhow? Are you really this much of a jerk, or do you just think it's cool to trash your boss and say words like 'dyke?'"

Sounding defensive, Troy says, "I just mean that it will be different with a woman in charge. She'll favor other women and try to play tough-ass with the guys. Before you know it, she'll start promoting women ahead of men, wear her hair in a bun, and smoke cigars."

Lou laughs.

"I'm serious. We already got a pool going to see how many days it takes before her hair goes on top of her head or she cuts it butch style," says Troy, with a strong emphasis on the word "butch" simply to irritate Chris and me.

"A buck says ten days," Lou spits out. "Make that two bucks!"

Again, the temptation to leave the table is almost overpowering. But, at the same time, I'm intrigued by what these guys might say next. It's kind of like slowing down to look at a train wreck. You don't really want to look, but at the same time, you don't want to miss something horrific. You know, like watching the scary parts of a movie with your hands in front of your face and your fingers spread wide apart.

Seeing the look on my face, Lou quickly adds, "Oh, relax, Tom. We're just havin' a little fun. I'm sure Betty will be fine. It's just gonna be different working for a gal, that's all—different."

"How so?" I ask. "In what way?"

"I don't know," says Lou, uncomfortable with the question. "You know, like we gotta watch our language, and maybe dress a little neater—stuff like that.

"Yeah," says Troy, revving up again, "watch her cut off the balls of the first guy who tries to get in her way."

"That means you're safe, Princess," says Lou with a wink and a feigned lisp.

"I'm curious," I say as we all ignore Lou. "Do you think that women are incapable of leadership or do you just hate all women?" The question is asked with a smile as well as a tone of concern.

"Jesus Christ, I don't hate women, Tom," Troy quickly defends himself. "I just prefer taking my orders from a guy. Harvey knew this business and how to treat people. You could talk to him, have a beer, shoot the shit. You know—guy stuff."

Chris joins in, "So, what makes you think you can't do that with Betty? She's smart, been here forever, and works her tail off."

"I'm just telling you that I agree with Lou, that's all. It's gonna be different without the old man."

"Give her a chance," I add. "She may surprise you. And, Troy, do yourself a favor, check your attitude and hold your comments down—at least pull back on the personal assassination stuff. You may not like her style and she may not be one-of-the-guys, but she's dedicated to this company and won't tolerate anything or anyone that doesn't advance the corporate bottom line."

I continue, "Personally, as much as I loved the old man, I think she'll do a better job of running the day-to-day operations. And, she won't let the old-boy network or cronyism interfere with making tough decisions."

Silence and a quick look around the table tell me that I may have just crossed the line. Clearly—to these guys—my management stripes were showing and glowing.

Balancing the dual roles of "one-of-the-guys" and "McGregor from HR" has always been a bit of a challenge. A challenge, I admit, that at times still makes me uncomfortable. I believe that Lou and Troy trust that what is said at the table, bar, and ball field stays there, but there are moments when I give them pause. This is one of those moments. As for Chris, what is both infuriating and admirable is that he seemingly could care less about office politics. He always speaks his mind regardless of who is listening. This attitude wins both friends and enemies.

"But, Mr. McGregor, sir," says Troy with exaggerated deference, "isn't it that very same 'old-boy' network and cronyism that allowed Harvey to build this business?"

"Come on Troy, don't give me that 'Mr. McGregor' stuff," I say with exasperation in my voice. "And, yes, the old-boy network did allow Harvey to start this plant, no question about it. That was the way things were back then. However, once established, it took results to keep the customers happy and to show a profit. And to do that, Harvey was smart enough to hire good people. Betty was one of the first."

In a much more relaxed tone I continue, "If you respect Harvey and what he stood for, respect the fact that Betty was his personal choice to succeed him. She always gets the job done, and for Harvey that is—or rather was—the bottom line. He was never a fool when it came to business."

"Okay," says Lou, "speaking of bosses, what's the difference between a mosquito and a boss?…One's a relentless, pain-inflicting bloodsucker. The other's an insect."

We all smile.

Taking this opportunity, I apologize for my mini-lecture to Troy. Not because I didn't mean what I said, but for the fact that it came off as either a "Respect your elders" shot or a warning missive from management.

"Troy, I'm sorry for sounding like an old man or a stooge from the front office. That's not the case, and I think you all know it. I think, in part, it's still the shock of losing Harvey. Also, while Betty's not the warmest person, I know from working side-by-side with her for all these years that she really is the right person for the job. And, she's very nice, as well. It's just that you won't see that side very often. Maybe in part because she is a woman, she feels she has to come across a bit more sternly. Otherwise, you clowns won't take her seriously."

I can see from Troy's quick head nod and tilt that all is well.

Chris jumps in, "I think we're all due a little blow-off time. Everybody's a little anxious about what may happen now that there's a new boss. I, for one, am going to take the kids and head for the lake this weekend. An hour and a half of softball on Thursday nights followed by a quick beer is not what I would call putting balance in my life."

With a round of "Amen," and the sound of Lou trying to get off one more one-liner, we push away from the table and head back to our stations.

What Would Mickey Say?
About Leadership and Men at Work

Tom: Professional athletics isn't exactly what I would call "normal" work, Mick. Can you relate at all to what these guys are talking about?

Mickey: Well, not about working for a woman, but, yeah, some of it. I sure know what it's like to work for a jerk and what it's like to be around leaders. I spent time with both.

Tom: So, who was the jerk and who were the leaders and what made them that way?

Mickey: As a Yankee, I worked for Casey, Ralph Houk, Yogi, Johnny Keane, and then Ralph again. Of course, Casey sticks out more than the rest because he was the first, and I spent ten years with him. They were all good, I guess, in their own way, otherwise they wouldn't have gotten to manage the Yankees. It's just that they all had their own style and it worked with some of us and not with the rest.

Tom: Who worked best for you, Mick, and how would you describe their style?

Mickey: Let me take them each one by one and see if it answers your question.

Now, you have to remember that Casey was like a father to me—actually, more like a grandfather—in the early years. I was just nineteen when I came to New York and Casey was sixty. My dad was only thirty-seven.

Casey used to call me "son" and "kid" and put his arm around me when he was giving me advice. I can't say that he taught me a whole lot about baseball, but he sure knew how to get the best out of me. The book on Casey was that he was great with young ballplayers and when I started in 1951, we had whole bunch of them. He'd yell at us for screwing up, but he gave us room to grow and he let a lot of things slide.

I remember once when Billy Martin, Whitey Ford, and I decided to take a side trip to Kentucky for some fun after an exhibition game in Cincinnati. We lost track of the time and ended up missing the team train to Pittsburgh. So we decide to just spend the night, party some more, and catch a plane in the morning. Well, it snows like hell all night and all the flights are cancelled. We end up paying $500 for a cab and drive five-and-a-half hours to the ballpark. We get there just as the other guys are running on the field to take batting practice. Casey notices that we are missing and comes looking for us in the locker room. Meanwhile, we are scrambling to get dressed and I'm looking down, tying my shoes, and jabbering away to Billy. The only problem is that Billy's not there—he's in the can. When I look up, Casey is standing over me looking pissed as hell. He knows something is up but isn't quite sure what. He cusses a blue streak and stomps out yelling that Billy and I are going to play every single inning of the game. We feel like hell after partying all night, no sleep, and 300 miles in a car, but we hit the field feeling lucky that all we got was a tongue whooping. Casey knows we're suffering, but this is his way of delivering a message.

Well, at my first at bat, I hit a monster of a home run over the grandstand. Casey just shakes his head and says, "Nice hit, Mickey. Take the rest of the day off." As I head for the corner of the dugout to take a nap, I hear Billy singing, "Teacher's pet, teacher's pet!"

Probably the best picture of Casey and how he related to the young players was in a cartoon that appeared in the New York papers. It showed the three of us, Billy, Whitey, and me, in front of Casey, who's sitting high up on a platform looking like a judge or a school principal. We look repentant as we take our medicine, but in our back pockets tucked almost out of sight are slingshots, BB guns, and peashooters—ready for action just as soon as we're finished getting yelled at.

I think I got off easiest because I was always more of a follower than a leader. No question about it, Billy was the leader with Whitey a close second. They were stubborn, strong-willed, and always had a twinkle in their eyes. For the most part, I was just having fun, following along, and enjoying the ride. It's kinda like what the professor said earlier about peer influence being stronger than parents. Casey was the dad, but Billy and Whitey were my buddies. I cared more about what they thought than about what Casey said.

Tom: And your other bosses, Ralph Houk, Yogi, and Johnny Keane?

Mickey: Ralph was great. A real field-general, solid in his knowledge, disciplined without bullying, and respectful of a player's ability. Ralph treated his players like they were adults and never questioned their ability. If a player had a tough string of games, he wouldn't scold and give fatherly advice, like Casey did; Ralph would just tell you not to get too discouraged—to hang in there and continue to do the best you could. Ralph got the best out of his players because they respected him and trusted his leadership. Under Ralph in 1961, we set a new Yankee record for wins and ran away with the pennant. That was also the year Roger and I chased Ruth's record for single-season homers. Roger broke the record with sixty-one and I hit fifty-four.

I think that part of my success in '61 was because, at the beginning of the season, Ralph pulled me aside and made me team captain. I was expecting the customary opening day lecture about behaving myself, but instead he gave me the responsibility of leading the team. When I asked him how I was supposed to do that, he said I was simply to lead by example. I was one of the veterans and the others would look to me for leadership. Nobody had ever done that before—made me accountable and responsible for the success of a team. I liked it and took it seriously. For the first time as a ballplayer, I took the focus off me and placed it on the team. Of course, it helped that the press was making Roger out to be the bad guy and me the good guy, but Ralph managed that well, also. People thought Roger and I were enemies that year, but it just wasn't so. In fact, we were quite close and Ralph had a lot to do with that.

I wish people along the way had given me more responsibility and held me more accountable for things. I think that if I'd had the right mentor when I first came up, I could have been a great leader—I really do. Like Babe Ruth, I had hoped to stay in baseball all my life, to be a coach or maybe even a manager. But, like Ruth, nobody ever took me seriously. After I retired, the Yankees hired me as their first base coach, but quickly it became very clear that all they wanted me for was to bring people to the ballpark. They wanted to parade me around like a circus monkey. Management never seriously thought of me as a real coach. And, who could blame them? Most of my career, I played for one person—Mickey Mantle—and gave little thought to the rest of my team. Well, maybe I played for two people—my dad, Mutt Mantle, and me.

In all honesty, I just wasn't a leader. Like I said, I think I could have been, but I wasn't. I used to wonder why Billy became a successful manager; after all, he was worse off the field than I was. The difference between us was that Billy hated to lose—period. Regardless how well or poorly he personally did, he hated for the team to lose. He would sacrifice his own stats if it meant the team would win. Besides, like I also said, Billy was a leader. He had charm, charisma, a sense of purpose, and a forceful personality. People felt confident in his presence and gladly let him lead, even if it didn't seem to make sense or sometimes his antics led to trouble.

In his eighteen seasons as a manager, Billy won six pennants for four different teams and won three World Series. He was volatile and a little crazy, but nobody questioned his desire to win.

Tom: How about Yogi and Johnny Keane?

Mickey: Well, Johnny Keane may have been the National League Manager of the Year in '64, but he wasn't right for the Yankees in 1965. Under him, we took a nosedive and went from first place in '64 to sixth place in '65. He was a drill sergeant who was arrogant, dictatorial, and standoffish. Everything was to be done his way. No drinking, no late nights, and no dissension. His way—period.

He and I rarely talked, but we did have some serious staring contests. I was miserable as my batting average slipped from .303 in 1964 to .255 in '65. My home runs dropped from thirty-five to nineteen. If I had been in better financial shape, I would have retired at the end of the season. In fact, both Roger and I were ready to call it quits or hope for a trade. For Roger, the breaking point came when Keane tried to force him to play with a broken wrist.

As for me, I almost came to blows with him on a number of occasions. One of Keane's ways of punishing me for drinking or staying out past curfew was to send me to center field for a grueling hour or so of fungo. Now, having been the starting center fielder for the American League All Stars every year since 1952, I had a pretty good idea how to play the position, so this was just his way of showing everyone who was boss. The idea was to punish and humiliate me in front of the team. One time, after close to an hour of running my butt all over the field, he hit a shallow pop-up. I ran, caught it, and in the same motion, threw a bullet at his head. He ducked, but I think he got the point.

Now, don't get me wrong, Tom. I'm not saying that I was guiltless and Keane was just out to get me. Far from it. As I remember, I was quite a handful that year. It's just that his way of dealing with me—punishment and humilia-tion—clearly was not working, and instead of trying a different approach, he just got more heavy handed.

Yogi came in right before Keane and was the opposite. He was named manager in 1964 because Ralph Houk was bumped up to the front office to replace Roy Haney as the vice president and general manager of the Yankees.

Yogi was a gentle soul who had a hard time not being just one of the guys. He had been a player with most of us for so long that he couldn't bring himself to make demands. He would just nicely remind us to follow the rules and then turn his back when we broke them. The problem was that the younger guys like Tom Tresh, Phil Linz, and Joe Pepitone would see this and act just like us veterans. They liked Yogi, but had little respect for his authority.

We won the American League pennant that year but lost the World Series in seven games to the St. Louis Cardinals. Johnny Keane managed the Cardinals. Yogi got fired and Keane was hired as the Yankee Manager.

Okay, one more Yogi quote. After a long hitless spell, a reporter asks Yogi when he expects to break out of his slump. "Slump?" asks, Yogi. "Hell, I ain't in no slump, I just ain't hitting."

The Professor Speaks
About Leadership and Men at Work

Tom: It seems that each month, Professor, there is a new book about lead-ership. We look to everyone from Attila the Hun to former NYC Mayor, Rudy Guiliani, for guidance. What are your thoughts? How important is leadership and what should we look for in a leader?

Professor Edwards: Before I give you a detailed read on men and lead-ership, let me give you an example of the relationship between Mantle and Stengel. In 1958, Casey was called on to testify before the Senate Subcommittee on antitrust and monopoly.

Senator Kefauver, the presiding officer, played it square, as he did every-thing else, starting with his simple request that ol' Case, who never did anything simply, briefly establish his background: "Mr. Stengel," he began, "you are the manager of the New York Yankees. Will you give us very briefly your background and views about this legislation?"

Forty-five minutes later, the water was muddier than at the dawn of creation. This is how Casey explained how major league managers are made and unmade:

"Well, I started in professional baseball in 1910.... I had many years that I was not so successful as a ballplayer, as it is a game of skill. And then I was no doubt discharged by baseball, in which I had to go back to the minor leagues as a manager. I became a major league manager in several cities and was discharged. We call it discharged because there was no question that I had to leave...."

At some point, Senator Kefauver tried to get Casey back on target: "Mr. Stengel, I am not sure that I made my question clear...."

"Well, that's all right," replied Casey, "I'm not sure I'm going to answer clearly, either."

"I am asking you, sir," continued Kefauver, "why it is that baseball wants this bill passed?"

What Casey said continues to bring smiles to all who recall his words:

"I would say I would not know, but I would say the reason they want it passed is to keep baseball going as the highest paid ball sport that has gone into baseball, and from the baseball angle—I am not going to speak of any other sport. I am not here to argue about these other sports. I am in the baseball business. It has been run cleaner than any business that was ever put out in the one hundred years at the present time...."

Completely befuddled, Senator Kefauver turns to Mickey and asks: "Mr. Mantle, do you have any observations with reference to the applicability of the antitrust laws to baseball?"

Mickey, true to his skipper, simply smiled in his country-boy, ah-shucks manner and replied, "My views are just about the same as Casey's."

At that point, the laughter could no longer be contained and their part of the hearing adjourned shortly thereafter.

Tom: Not to beat a cliché to death, but "the blind leading the blind" does come to mind.

Professor Edwards: Tom, it is our nature to seek guidance, security, and strength from others, to look outside ourselves for glimpses of the future and for reinforcement that we are on the right track. Small children look to their parents and teachers; adolescents look to their peers, sports heroes, TV, music, and other forms of popular media. As adults, some people seek mentors, ask questions, and pay attention as they work toward independent thinking, while others remain forever under the controlling influence of a boss, a spouse, a parent, alcohol, drugs, or whatever trend and attitude currently holds the nation's attention and scores high in popularity.

As an example of how we seek out and respond to leaders, there was a perfect case that happened during the 2003 summer blackout in New York City. When all the traffic lights went out, movement was coming to a chaotic stop when a young man on a bicycle decided to take action. With no traffic control experience, he placed himself in the center of a major intersection and took control. With confidence and clear motions, he moved traffic east and west while he held back the north- and south-bound lanes. After a reasonable amount of time, he reversed the flow and continued in this manner until a "real" traffic cop showed up. People responded because they needed someone to take control. They readily and thankfully followed the first person who presented a sense of authority and competence.

Mickey, for most of his life, was looking for guidance from others. He looked, first, to his dad and grandfather, then to Casey, Billy, Whitey, and anyone else who kept him from having to think too hard or work too hard to come up with answers all on his own. It didn't matter that Casey was speaking gibberish or that Billy was telling him things that he knew to be wrong or dangerous. Their tone and actions spoke with assurance and authority. Right up to the eighteen months before he died, he was just a kid who wanted nothing more than to play ball and have a good time. Whoever was leading in that direction was fine with him and when he couldn't find a person, the booze was a powerful and seductive replacement.

You see, Tom, leadership is at the core of who we are and who we see ourselves becoming. Hopes, dreams, self-esteem, success, failure, perseverance, and defeat all hinge on leadership. Leaders, good and bad—and don't forget the Hitlers, Stalins, and Saddam Husseins of this world—impact our lives in every way—physically, spiritually, and emotionally.

Tom: I understand what you're saying in the broad sense about parents, politicians, teachers, and spiritual leaders, but what about at work?

Professor Edwards: I don't care if you work in center field at Yankee Stadium or Joe's Machine Shop down on Main Street, U.S.A., your boss and whoever signs your paycheck has a huge impact on your life. That's why leadership is so important. Certainly there is no one leadership style that fits everyone's needs, but there are certain things that all good leaders have in common.

Tom: And?

Professor Edwards: At the risk of way over-simplifying this, here they are.

A Good Leader:
• gathers the facts and never shoots from the hip
• takes care of his mind, body, and spirit
• has a sense of purpose
• is his own person
• listens, clarifies, and listens some more
• gets close...but not too close to workers
• sweats the small stuff
• begs, borrows, and steals great ideas
• has precision focus
• uses every bit of life experience—the good, bad, and truly ugly

chapter
twelve

All Jammed up in the Sandwich Generation
Raising Kids and Taking Care of Aging Parents

We find out at lunch why Jim has, again, missed so many days of work. No sooner had his daughter, Shelley, settled down when his live-in mother-in-law took a turn for the worse. Her need for long-term care is such that Jim and his wife can no longer keep her at home. The stress of raising teenagers, dealing with menopause/andropause, and an aging parent has taken a serious toll on Jim. His saving grace is that now he is talking about it and asking for help.

His teammates at the table offer Jim advice. Some valuable, some pretentious, and some just plain awful. But, the group is responding like a team. They are truly trying to help one another.

Jim begins to feel better and expresses his appreciation to the guys. Not an easy thing for a man to do. Lou makes it a bit easier with—you guessed it—mother-in-law jokes.

Mickey talks about how he deferred all of the family responsibility to Merlyn and the guilt it created toward the end of his life. He also speaks about a sense of isolation felt in that sea of adulation.

Using a popular (but, bizarre) sitcom family, the professor gives advice on how to avoid the dangers that come with being a member of the "Sandwich Generation."

"So, okay, Jim," says Troy, "what's the mystery? Where you been, man? God knows you're not the greatest first baseman, but you're sure as hell better than Connellan! He couldn't catch a ball if you rolled it to him."

"Personal." That's all Jim says. "Personal."

"Well," continues Troy, "just tell us if you can't make the last two games. I'll recruit my grandmother rather than put Connellan back in the lineup. I bet in Little League he was the kid they stuck in right field to pick flowers and chase bugs."

"All right," says Lou as he hauls his wagon of grease, fat, and sugar to the table, "here's a simple baseball joke for a table of simple baseball guys."

Everyone turns to look as Lou approaches. You can feel the mood of the group elevate every time he shows up.

Have you ever noticed how some guys change the mood of a room simply by showing up? All these Friday lunch guys do that.

Take Troy for example. He's like driving past the scene of an accident. You're both excited and repelled when you see it approaching. Against your better judgment you look, but always feel guilty and a bit queasy after you pass by. Just the same, you know you'll look again.

Chris is another of those approach/avoid kind of guys. Because of his intelligence, passion, and honesty, you're glad to see him, but his welcome wears thin once the arrogance and know-it-all finger wagging takes over.

Jim is like a bucket of lukewarm water. His cynical approach to life brings out the natural complainer in all of us—at times we all need to wail—but he can sure bring a group down. You want to support him and kick his butt at the same time.

Ted is something else. His glibness, Eddie Haskell-like charm, and rule-bending appeals to our adolescent desire to hang out with an outlaw. You're attracted to his rogue behavior while, at the same time, he makes your skin crawl. He's like a bad habit: you know he's dangerous, but you can't seem to pull away. When you finally do (or when the "bad habit" gets fired…), you wonder what the attraction was in the first place and why you didn't turn away years ago.

And then…there's Lou—a fine blend of innocence, court jester, and sage. You know that there's more to Lou than he reveals, and, to be honest, you're grateful not to know more. Every group needs comic relief. We're blessed with Lou. He's kind of a John Goodman meets Steinbeck's Lennie from *Of Mice and Men*.

I guess, if I am going to pigeonhole guys at the table, I need to find a place for me. Probably the most accurate words used to describe my impact on a group's mood are "comfort" and "security." No surprises, excitement, highs, or lows. Pretty much like a rudder that keeps a small boat on a steady course. Every once in awhile, I would like to veer into the high winds and open seas but the twin sisters of reason, Prudence and Caution, keep me locked in the safety zone. I guess that's what attracts me to the other guys in the group. Through each of them, I get to feel what it's like to take risks. Pretty sad, actually.

With a big grin and a fist full of French fries, Lou begins.

"A man walks into a bar with a dog. The bartender says, 'You can't bring that dog in here.' 'You don't understand,' says the man. 'This is no regular dog—he can talk.' 'Listen, pal,' says the bartender. 'If that dog can talk, I'll give you a hundred bucks.' The man puts the dog on a stool, and asks him, 'What's on top of a house?' 'Roof!' 'Right. And what's on the outside of a tree?' 'Bark!' 'And who's the greatest baseball player of all time?' 'Ruth!'

"'I guess you've heard enough,' says the man. 'I'll take the hundred in twenties.' The bartender is furious. 'Listen, pal,' he says, 'get out of here before I belt you.'

"As soon as they're on the street, the dog turns to the man and says, 'Do you think I should have said DiMaggio?'"

Part of the fun of Lou's jokes is seeing how much he enjoys telling them. You get the feeling that he is really his own audience—you are simply there to keep people from thinking he's crazy.

"We had to put Mildred's mother in a nursing home," says Jim.

"What?" asks Lou.

"Evergreen Acres. We put her in Evergreen Acres out on M-51."

Everybody stops and looks at Jim. Not more than a word or two since his blowup a few weeks ago, and now he's volunteering information. Nobody really knows what to say.

"How old is she, Jim?" I finally break the silence.

"Christ, she must be 110," Jim says. "Or, maybe it just feels like she's been living with us for that long. She's only eighty-three—after filling out a million forms, I should know that, by now.

"I tell you something, between my kid taking drugs, Millie's menopause, getting passed over for that promotion, and dealing with a sick mother-in-law, I've had it. No more. I'm going nuts. Spatalie, old friend, here I come!"

His reference to Spatalie's suicide is said with enough lightness so as not to create alarm. But, still, you get the sense that this is not a new thought.

I ask, "So how's Shelley doing? Is rehab working out?" As I ask the questions I realize how troubled Jim really must be. After all, if I have to distract him from thoughts of suicide by asking about his drugged-out teenager, things are seriously wrong in his life. Throw in a wife in menopause, a dead-end to your career, aging, and a sick mother-in-law that you never liked, and…well, you get the picture. All of a sudden the entire table begins to lend support.

"I saw Shelley the other day at the mall," adds Troy. "She looked great. And, trust me, I know what zombie chicks look like—she's clean," he says with the assurance of an expert. "So were the kids that she was with."

"Yeah, she said she saw you. Of course," he adds with a hint of a smile, "I told her to never speak to you and run like hell if you ever get near her." This is the first smile any of us have seen in weeks—make that months. "She's really doing much better. Thanks for asking."

"She's over twelve, Jimbo," says Lou. "That makes her too old for Troy, here, anyway."

Jim laughs.

Chris picks up on Jim's shifting mood, "Hey, Jim, how does it feel having Mildred's mom out of the house?"

"Well, it was a difficult decision—for Mildred, not for me—but now that it's done, I think we're all going to feel better—even Lucille, Mildred's mom." Jim adds, "She was miserable these past few months. All of us were. We just didn't know it."

Seeing an opening, Lou shoots, "Damn, boy! You should've asked us. We would have told you that you were miserable!"

Not letting go of the reins, Lou plows ahead, "One day two old ladies were standing outside the nursing home casually having a smoke," he begins. "After being outside for awhile it started to rain on them. Suddenly, one of the ladies took out a condom, cut off the tip, and slipped it over her cigarette. The other lady asked, 'What's that for?' The first replied, 'It's to keep my cigarette dry when I'm outside smoking and it starts to rain.' The second lady said, 'That's a pretty crafty idea.'

"The following day the old lady went to the drugstore to get some condoms. She walked in and told the clerk, 'I'd like some condoms please.' The clerk looked at the old lady, rather baffled at why she would need condoms. However, he asked, 'What brand would you like, Madam?' The old lady smiled and replied, 'I don't care what brand you give me, as long as it fits a Camel.'"

Visibly relaxing, Jim sits back in chair and replies with a laugh, "Hell, swap the Marlboro Man for that Camel and you just described Lucille!"

I think about my own situation. Laurie's an only child and with her mom gone and Bill, my father-in-law, getting up there, I know we will have to deal with this issue before we know it. "Was it difficult finding a good place for her?"

"A nightmare, at first," says Jim. "The whole thing was somewhat scary, frightening, depressing, and confusing. Lucille doesn't have any money so we have to depend totally on Medicaid and Medicare to pay the bills. Once you do this, you are at the mercy of the state."

"They're all pretty much the same, aren't they?" asks Troy.

"No way!" shouts Chris. "There are new standards for quality and for patients' rights, but monitoring is difficult and enforcement is minimal. The less scrupulous homes risk paying fines rather than incur the cost of complying with regulations."

"Well, we have her in a pretty nice place, now. But it took a few days to get her settled. Lucille is perfectly lucid. Her mind is sharp as a tack—it's her lungs that are shot. Also the medicine to help her breathe is causing bone loss, so she's constantly getting fractures. That's why we can't keep her at home anymore— she needs constant care.

"After talking to a number of people and visiting all the area homes that take Medicare patients, Evergreen came out on top. Problem was that they didn't have any room, so they sent her to one of their other local homes. The one on Cherry Street."

Troy jerks his head up, "You mean the looney bin next to the old General Hospital? Whoa, talk about nut cases! When I was a kid, we used to dare each other to go inside. It was scarier than sneaking into Lynn's Funeral Parlor to look at the stiffs. I thought that place was just for wackos!"

"Why, Troy," says Chris with feigned sincerity, "I never realized you were so sensitive to the pain and suffering of others. I'm very impressed. Tell me, did you make fun of these poor souls and disturb grieving friends and relatives before or after you and your buddies pulled the wings off of flies and fried ants with a magnifying glass?"

"Before *and* after," says Troy with a broad grin and a fixed stare. "Then we went over to the park on First Street and harassed the prostitutes and beat up the winos. But, don't worry, Lycra Boy, we never bothered your mom and dad."

"All right, all right," says Lou. "Speaking of mothers, I heard that Troy's mother was once in a nursing home and she used to walk up and down the halls lifting her skirt while yelling, 'Supersex, supersex, supersex!' One day she walks up to this old guy recently admitted to the home. He's just sitting in his wheel-chair watching TV when all of a sudden she lifts her dress and starts yelling, 'Supersex! Supersex! Supersex!' The old guy looks away from the TV, gives her a quick once-over and quietly says, 'I believe I'll have the soup, thank you.'"

What Would Mickey Say?
About Raising Kids and Taking Care of Parents

Tom: Mickey, any advice on how to raise kids and take care of aging parents?

Mickey: Tom, you've got to be kidding. Asking me for advice on how to take care of anyone is like asking Yogi and Casey to debate the meaning of life: you'll get a lot of words, but it won't make much sense.

Tom: Give it a try.

Mickey: Well, first of all, I have to repeat myself and tell men the same thing I tell boys. Don't be like me. Don't take your kids drinking with you. Don't live your life for your dad or anyone else. Don't set a bad example by cheating on your kids' mom and having the kids cover for you. Don't think you can make up for real affection by buying your mom stuff but never really spending time with her.

Tom: Any more "Don'ts?"

Mickey: Yeah, don't forget that your kids look up to you and model their lives on how you live yours. Don't forget that someday you'll be old and it will be pretty lonely if you never see your kids, or if they show up only because they feel obligated or sorry for you. And, one more, if you live your life like I did, don't think things won't happen to you like they happened to me. Odds are, they will.

Tom: Lots of "Don'ts," how about some "Dos"?

Mickey: Okay. But keep in mind that most of this advice comes from someone who learned too late.

If I could do it again, here's a partial list of things I would do if I had the chance:

- Hug my boys often and teach them that it's okay to cry and show fear
- Respect my dad, but find my own voice
- Be patient with my mom and give us both a chance to know each other
- Think about what I say and what I do, knowing that my boys will question their own thoughts and actions side-by-side with mine
- Tell them all that I love them. And, tell them a whole bunch of times.

Not too fancy but that's about it. I guess it boils down to being honest and open about feelings while accepting and appreciating other people and life. Like I said, not too fancy.

The Professor Speaks
About Raising Kids and Taking Care of Parents

Tom: We hear a lot about the so-called "sandwich generation," Professor—people like Jim who are both raising kids and caring for parents. What advice do you have?

Professor Edwards: The challenges of the sandwich generation are here to stay and they will become an increasingly significant part of our lives in the years to come. For some SGs (members of the sandwich generation, usually between forty and sixty years of age), this can mean high-level enrichment as they learn from the wisdom of their aging parents, and the innocence and vitality of their children, and—in increasing numbers—their grandchildren. However, for others, the challenges will not only crush opportunities for enrichment, they will also destroy families.

Tom: How do you keep from getting all jammed up in the sandwich generation? How do you avoid getting crushed?

Professor Edwards: There are many variations of the SG dilemma, but for our purposes today, let's create a fictitious household. We will call them the Addams Family.

Under the same roof there's Father Gomez, Mother Morticia, Grandmama Addams, Uncle Fester, and the little ones, Wednesday and Pugsley. There's also cousin Itt, but he's a family secret. (We all have at least one, don't we?) And, like any typical American family, there is an assortment of pets, including the family Lion, Kitty Kat; Pugsley's octopus, Aristotle; Wednesday's spider, Homer; and Morticia's childhood pet vultures, Hubert and Henry. Morticia's mother, Grandmother Frump, is pushing ninety, but for some reason prefers to live by herself in her own home, far away from the rest of the family.

Tom: Now, wait a minute, Professor....

Professor Edwards: I know, I know. Just humor me and pay attention, Tom.

Here's the background on the Addams family. They are a very loving extended family, or, at least, they used to be. They live at 001 Cemetery Lane in a lovely, quiet subdivision. In addition to family members living in the cemetery, there are many other colorful relatives that live close by, including Cousin Creep. Actually, Cousin Creep is a sad story. Pugsley accidentally zapped him with a disintegrator ray gun. Uncle Fester remembers, "There he was, giggling and laughing. Suddenly, there he wasn't—still giggling and laughing. It was kind of eerie."

Tom: Professor…?

Professor Edwards: Okay, sorry. Lou's influence is taking over. At any rate, let's use the Addams family to look at typical situations faced by today's SG.

Both Morticia's Uncle Fester and Grandmama Addams are showing signs of aging. They are forgetful, slower than they used to be, and both are dealing with chronic disease. Uncle Fester has diabetes, probably from too many sugar-coated bats and rides in the hearse when he could have easily walked. Grandma has arthritis, aggravated, no doubt, by living in the fruit cellar. They don't mean to be a burden, but increasingly they require medical attention and seem needier at home. Besides expensive healthcare (every year the prescription co-pay increases and more treatments are denied by Medicare), the seniors have special diets, need barrier-free accommodations, and require extra preparation time when the family travels beyond Cemetery Lane. In addition, Grandma Frump recently fell and nearly broke her hip. It's clear that she should not be living alone, but she is so independent and stubborn that nobody wants to bring up the subject of moving her into the big house or, possibly, moving her to a nursing home. This puts an added burden on Morticia, who since the fall feels an obligation to stop by at least once each day.

Meanwhile, the kids are constantly being teased at school because of their unique heritage and strange customs (the community is mostly comprised of Methodists). Wednesday is beginning to withdraw from her family, and Pugsley is becoming a behavior problem at school (something about threatening to turn Rodney Summers into a toad). Mr. Karloff, the school counselor, says that the children are being neglected and need more parental guidance and supervision.

Morticia and Gomez are at their wits' end. While neither will talk much about it, they blame the other's relatives for the problems at school and for the growing tension in their marriage. A once red-hot sex life is all but over, and they seldom talk except to argue about money. Morticia feels trapped and Gomez feels like a failure.

The sad part is that this is really a loving family with good intentions. Gomez and Morticia love their aging relatives and they are devoted parents. They are also devoted to each other. She used to call him "Bubala" and "Mon Cheri." He used to call her "Cara Mia" and "Cara Bella." Now they call each other names that…well, names that would make Uncle Fester blush and at a volume that would wake the dead—in fact, it probably has. They just don't know what to do.

In their quiet personal moments, each of them wishes that everyone would just GO AWAY and give them some peace. Of course, as soon as they begin to feel sorry for themselves, they are overcome with pangs of guilt and remorse and vow—once again—to make the best of a bad situation. Unfortunately, they don't have a clue what that means.

Tom: So, what do they do?

Professor Edwards: First, let's break this down and take a look at the issues for each generation. Before you can ever hope to solve a problem you have to first identify what the problem is. Here are the issues, as I see them, for the Addams family and for other families just like them. Well…maybe not just like them.

Let's look at the kids, Pugsley and Wednesday, first. Like all kids, they want independence, love, acceptance, and respect. They are embarrassed by their parents, at times, but will fight anyone who trashes their family. The kids think that Uncle Fester and Grandmama Addams are somewhat strange with their old customs and styles, but feel genuine affection for them. Of course, they often resent all the attention given to the seniors, but for the most part they grin and bear it.

Uncle Fester and Grandma are really more like the children than they are like Gomez and Morticia. Like the kids, they want, need, and expect a lot of attention and often feel hurt and slighted if they are not the center of activity. They also feel, at times, that they are a burden to their children and, in their darker moments, wish perhaps that the end would hurry up and get here. They are concerned about declining health, limited funds, and having to depend so heavily upon their children. Yes, certainly, they enjoy time with the kids and appreciate what Gomez and Morticia have done for them, but still they miss people their own age and long for the days when they had the body, spirit, and means to live independently.

As for Gomez and Morticia, they just want HELP! They want to feel appreciated; they need someone to take the pressure off of them; they need and want more support from each other (there can never be too much), and they want to again feel sexual heat and passion for each other. Morticia wants to know when it's "my turn," and Gomez is afraid of getting old and missing his chance to be on top of the world.

Tom: Of course, there are challenges for everyone, but what, specifically, can Gomez do? Or, any man, for that matter?

Professor Edwards: Well, how about this. Here are five ways men can avoid getting jammed up in the sandwich generation:

1. Me First! On the surface, this may seem selfish, but it is critical for all the Gomezs out there and Morticias too.

When you fly in an airplane with small children, what does the flight attendant tell you to do if the cabin pressure falls and the oxygen masks drop? You're instructed to secure your mask first and then your child's. Unless and until you are safe, secure, and strong, you are no good to anyone else. It is critical that you take time to relax and keep physically fit. Even if you can only steal away as little as thirty minutes each day.

When time is a real crunch, consider blending your exercise and relaxation. A quiet, reflective walk after dinner is one way. Or, listening to your favorite music while on an exercise bike. Mindless TV works for some, but for others, it's only another form of procrastination leading to more stress and guilt. If you have a favorite show that really grabs you, great. Sit, watch, and enjoy. But, beware of inertia—things at rest tend to stay at rest!

2. Nurture your relationship and your partner. If you're sharing this sandwich with a life partner, protect and support the relationship. We tend to fire off quickly around those with whom we feel most safe and secure. As a result, things are said, slights are made, and issues that need attention are put off until those free moments that never seem to appear. A hug, a wink, a smile, an affectionate pinch, a joke, and even a pleasant knowing shrug, goes a long way.

An honest and open mood check is also critical. This is no time to play martyr. If you need a break, say so. If you feel insecure in the relationship, say so. If you need sexual intimacy, say so. If you are afraid for the future, say so. But, remember, it works both ways. And, guys, we are not as dense as we sometimes wish to appear. Yes, we would like our partner to openly and verbally express feelings, but, be honest, there are times when we actually do get the non-verbals and "the code." Often, we clearly hear the message that comes with "I'm fine," followed by a whimper and a long sigh; the "No, nothing's wrong," that dangles without eye contact; and the long periods of silence that follow an argument. It's just easier to pretend we don't.

3. Make it a family sandwich. You know those long sub sandwiches, the ones that you slice up and share with a group? Well, think of this time of life as a family sandwich. Everyone—kids, parents, grandparents—shares in the joys, challenges, and responsibilities. Grandma needs to go to the doctor? No reason

why your driving-age kids can't take a turn. Got little ones at home who still need a sitter? Get Gramps to help out, if he can. They will both benefit. Tight on cash? Don't hesitate to have Mom and/or Dad help out, if they can. Same goes for the kids. Assuming full responsibility for the care and well being of your children and your parents will only wear you down and everyone will suffer. Share, learn, and enjoy.

4. No secrets. Who are you kidding? Do you really think the kids don't sense the tension in the house? When you speak in front of your parents about the problems your kids are having in school, do you actually think they don't hear you and feel bad, as well? When and if the time comes to consider long-term care for a parent, don't you believe it's crossed his or her mind, also? When people live together or have frequent contact, they develop a highly sensitive degree of group awareness. They know the feel of happiness; they can smell fear, and they understand the meaning behind subtle voice inflections. For close family members, a foot shake, a finger tap, a head turn, and a lip smack work like sophisticated weather station instruments. They can signal clear sailing or they can serve as a warning that there's a storm a brewin' and it's time to batten down the hatches. No secrets, please. Honest, open discussions using age-appropriate language for the kids and non-patronizing clarity for the old folks work like a charm.

5. Dignity and privacy for all. Unless you are living in the poorest of conditions, there is no reason not to give everyone their privacy. This goes for parents living on their own as well as for those living with you. For the live-in parents, this means having their own room. If the parents are still able to live in their own home, they are entitled to live their own life. I've often heard SGs ask their parents, "Where were you?" "Why didn't you call?" "Who are you spending time with?" and similar role-reversal questions. Certainly, if the parent has medical needs, the SGs need to check to make sure appointments are kept and medications are taken. However, beyond health and safety concerns, allow the parents to maintain as much dignity and independence as possible. Remember, once upon a time they changed your diaper.

Small children can share a room if need be, but once they approach the teen years, they, too, should have every opportunity to escape to their own sheltered space. And, it goes without saying that the SGs must also have a sanctuary where they can simply Be.

chapter
thirteen

One Ding Dong Too Many
Lou

*S*hock. *That's the only word—shock. But, of course, nobody should be shocked. It was winking and laughing right in front of us every day. For years, we made jokes, smiled, and affectionately shook our heads at its audacity, bigger-than-life presence, and sheer force of denial. How could something so deadly come wrapped in something so full of life, so gentle, so welcoming, so accepting, so, so...Lou.*

Right before last night's game, the Big Guy was sitting on the bench just rubbing and rubbing the side of his face. I know it was the left side because he rubbed with his mitt. He said it felt like he just got back from the dentist and the Novocain hadn't worn off, kind of a tingling, numb feeling.

At the plate, in the first inning, he kept blinking his eyes and stepping out of the batter's box. We thought he was just being Lou. You know, goofing off, pretending the pitcher was throwing the ball so fast he couldn't see it. When he struck out, everybody, and I mean EVERYBODY, howled with laughter—the greatest humiliation in slow-pitch softball is to strike out. Troy hollered something about getting his mother to pinch-hit for him. We should have known something was up when Lou didn't even smile. Lou is...was...is one of those guys who smiles at everything. Not a dull or stupid smile, but a smile that says, "I'm just like you—no need to get uncomfortable or try to impress me—I'm just like you...no better, no worse."

When he ran to left field in the bottom of the first he never even made it past third base. He tripped over his spikes (we laughed, again...), regained his balance, smothered his head in the same glove he used to rub his cheek, and then he fell to the ground. He just collapsed and went straight down. It was like some-one pulled the plug—full motion one moment and then...nothing.

Fortunately, the ball field is right next to the Township Hall and the fire station. Without CPR, they said he would have died before reaching the ER at St. Luke's. So, instead of being dead, he is lying in the Intensive Care Unit in a deep coma hooked up to machines that beep, whoosh, and click.

The talk at the table is, naturally, about Lou.

Mickey talks about living in the Village of Someday, and the shock of realizing that he would one day die. Of course, as he has since the beginning of his visits, he takes full responsibility for everything that happened to him.

The professor talks about comas and second chances.

Today is so very *wrong*. Different, strange, lonely, and frightening in a way that can only be felt, not explained. It's just very *wrong*. Nothing is as it was. And yet, everything is the same.

Harriett, a woman I've never seen when she wasn't wearing a blue hairnet, scoops and slings the same pasty-looking mashed potatoes she has for the past fifteen years. She greets everyone with the same question: "Want gravy with your taters?" And, just like most days, the UPS guy, Danny, is grabbing an apple and jogging out the door after delivering a package to our cafeteria manager, Roy. At the far corner table next to the candy machine, Jeff Griffith, Andy Joachim, and Ray Schmansky are arguing about which is a better place to watch a baseball game, Old Tiger Stadium or the new field over in Greek Town. Bruce Kingsbury complains about the cold potatoes and tasteless gravy.

Over by the salad bar, Judy Silverman drops a tray. People applaud and cheer. Embarrassed, Judy smiles and bows. Bobbie Niedermeyer just swears, grabs a mop, and starts to clean up the spilled milk....

I, or rather, we—Troy, Jim, Chris, and I—watch and listen from inside a virtual bubble. Everything we see past our table is distorted, dreamlike. Everything we hear—the words, clinking of silverware, shuffling of chairs, table chatter—sounds muffled and in some way obscene.

Scattered around the cafeteria, you see other small bubbles of Lou's friends slugging their way through this day. One holds the warehouse gang—Tommy

Todero, John Meyers, Suzie Farnham, and old Pete Palmer. Inside another bubble sits the rest of the softball team: Connellan, Revill, Millican, Runfola, and Powers. Every once in awhile one of them looks up from a full tray, shrugs his shoulders, and shakes his head as someone passes by asking the same question.

"So?" asks Troy as he sits down at our table, "any change?"

It seems sadly ironic that just a few weeks ago, Lou was asking me that same question about Harvey. "No," I reply, "he's still in a deep coma. I spoke with his mom this morning. It appears that the damage is worse than they originally thought. They aren't sure when, or if, he will regain consciousness."

"Whoa," says Troy.

Chris and Jim say nothing. They just look at me.

"What do you mean, 'if'?" asks Troy.

"The doctor told Mrs. Stevens that Lou suffered a massive brain stem stroke. This is the area of the brain that controls all of our involuntary, life-support functions, such as breathing rate, blood pressure, and heartbeat. They have him hooked up on machines to keep his heart beating and to keep him breathing."

Chris adds, "To keep it simple, Troy, a stroke is basically a sudden stop of blood flow to a part of the brain, which then kills brain cells. As a result, certain body functions may be impaired or lost."

This time, for some reason, we appreciate instead of resent Chris's air of authority as he continues. "In Lou's case, it's the part of his brain that tells his heart to beat and his lungs to breathe that was damaged."

"So he's a vegetable?" says Troy in a very Troy-like way. "Right? He's a vegetable? Lou's a friggin' vegetable?"

"Well, that's great, Troy. You continue to amaze me with your lack of sensitivity," says Chris.

"The fact is, there's still so much we don't know about how the brain compensates for the damage caused by stroke or brain attack. Some brain cells may be only temporarily damaged—not killed—and may resume functioning. In some cases, the brain can reorganize its own functioning. Sometimes, a region of the brain takes over for another region damaged by the stroke. Stroke survivors sometimes experience remarkable and unanticipated recoveries that can't be explained."

"What else did Lou's mom say?" asks Jim.

"She's scared that he's going to die," I tell the whole table. "Apparently, the next few hours will let the doctors better predict what will happen."

"So," Troy plows ahead, "you're saying he's either going to die or be a vegetable? I'd rather die." He seems oblivious to Chris's remark about sensitivity. "No way do I want someone to plug me into the wall so I can live. That's bullshit."

Jim speaks up. "First off, Troy, we don't have a clue what's going to happen so I suggest you just pray to whatever god will listen to you. That goes for all of us.

"Secondly," he continues, "put yourself in Lou's mom and dad's shoes, and then tell me how willing you are to pull the plug. No matter what anyone says, when it's your kid, you pray for a miracle. My God, they must be going crazy."

"I'm telling you, that if it was me lying up there with my brain fried, I'd want someone to pull the plug," says Troy. "I bet Lou feels the same way."

"You're nuts as well as insensitive," shouts Chris. "Lou enjoys life more than anyone I know. Right now, more than anything else, I bet he wishes he was biting into a big, thick steak or a greasy burger and washing it down with a cold beer. Hell, I'd gladly get it for him. I'd even listen to another of his stupid jokes."

"Tom," asks Jim, "did he draw up a Living Will or a Durable Power of Attorney?"

"I can't imagine that he did," I say. "No matter how much we encourage everyone to think about things like that, almost nobody does. I would be shocked if Lou had either one of those."

"What's a Living Will?" asks Troy.

"Technically, it's called an Advance Medical Directive," I explain. I don't know why, but I look at Chris for agreement and he nods. "It's a legal document that explains your healthcare wishes in the event of an emergency or terminal situation. You can make decisions about such things as CPR, feeding tubes, respirators, and other procedures designed to either get your heart beating again or keep you living.

"A Durable Power of Attorney for Healthcare is a document you sign that gives someone else the right to make healthcare decisions if you can't. That person is called a Patient Advocate."

"So, if I sign a piece of paper saying I don't want any tubes or wires or any of that stuff," says Troy, "nobody can put me in suspended animation?"

"Well," I say, "although most states have laws giving living wills legal force, our state has not yet passed such a law. Doctors and hospitals might comply with your wishes, but no one can provide absolute assurance."

"But," adds Jim, "the decisions of the Patient Advocate are legally binding. Mildred is the Patient Advocate for her mother, and I'm named as the backup advocate."

"That means," says Chris, "make sure you really like and trust your advocate because he is the one who has the power."

"Christ," says Troy, as he pushes himself back from the table and rubs his face. "I can't believe we're talking about this. There's no way I want to even think about this stuff. That's for old guys like you, Tom, and you, Jim. I just wanna do my job, collect my pay, and enjoy life."

Shaking his head, Chris says, "I told him, and told him, and told him. 'Lose the weight, quit smoking, cool it with the beer drinking, and knock off the burgers and salt!' I told him, I told him, I told him," he says again with his voice trailing off.

"Does it take something like this before you idiots get the message?" he adds in typical Chris fashion. He then looks with disgust at Troy's plate of French fries, my apple pie, and Jim's mashed potatoes and gravy.

"And he wonders why nobody shows up for his classes,"says Jim as Chris leaves the table.

"Okay, in honor of Lou," says Troy, "you guys wanna hear a joke?"

"No. No jokes, not today. "

What Would Mickey Say?
About Lou...

Tom: Mickey, any thoughts about Lou?

Mickey: Of course, it's very sad. I like Lou. He seems like a great guy who deserves better than this. It sounds like he didn't see it coming, the stroke and all.

Tom: Do you really think he didn't understand that all those cheeseburgers wouldn't catch up to him someday?

Mickey: I don't think that any guy really thinks that this stuff will happen to him. I heard all the talk about booze and diet and exercise, but figured it was for those other guys, not for me. Maybe I'm different, but I never really thought about the dying part of death. You know what I mean? I didn't think about getting sick. I just figured some day I would die. You know, just not wake up.

Tom: No, I'm not sure I know what you mean.

Mickey: Well, in my head at least, I was always going to be twenty years old. At some crazy level, I thought I would always be able to hit the ball a mile, run like the wind, and throw a rope from deep center to home. It's hard to explain, but until I saw pictures of myself after I got sick, and until I took a good look in the mirror, you know, right past my eyes and kind of like into my heart and soul, I didn't really think about the dying part of life and what I did to bring it on so fast. But, when it did hit me, the fact that I was dying and that I did this to myself, I felt a deep sadness in my heart, a punch in my gut, and a strange mix of both urgency and hopelessness. And, of course, I felt guilty for screwing everything up.

Tom: But, didn't you feel all this before you knew you were dying?

Mickey: Well, yeah, but until I got very close to the end, I figured I would have the time to fix everything. Knowing that I would be able to deal with it some other time gave me the permission to quit feeling bad, get drunk, and continue being a jerk. All I had to do was apologize and promise to start taking better care of myself…later.

Lou's not a stupid guy. He knew in his head that what he was doing wasn't right—the drinking and diet stuff, but I bet you a dozen glazed donuts that he also figured that someday he'd make changes. The only difference between him and me is that he might not get a chance to truly realize how short life is. Maybe that's a good thing.

Tom: Any advice?

Mickey: I can't remember where I heard this, but someone once said that the Village of Someday is a pretty crowded place, and the sooner you move out, the better. I kind of like that one.

The Professor Speaks
About Lou…

Tom: Professor?

Professor Edwards: Actually, Tom, Chris did a pretty good job of describing the medical side of Lou's condition. However, while we seem to know a lot about how the brain works and the dynamics of a stroke, we actually know very little. Every time we see a miracle recovery, like when someone comes out of a coma after months or even years, we realize that all we can do is speak in terms of relative severity and statistical predictability.

Tom: Meaning?

Professor Edwards: Meaning that we can only measure consciousness and ability using today's technology and we can only predict using yesterday's experience. As a simple example, think of the rate of infection prior to the discovery of microscopic bacteria. The killing bacteria were always there, we just couldn't see them. Once we did, the simple procedure of washing hands and keeping the operatory sterile saved thousands of lives. Also, think about artificial limbs, speech technology, and implants that let people, once thought of as permanently deaf, hear.

Tom: Are you saying that Lou may be more aware than we think he is?

Professor Edwards: Oh, without question. We can only measure what we can measure and, to sound even more confusing, we don't know what we don't know. At a level we can't measure, Lou may well hear, sense, and feel everything that's happening around him.

There are a number of instances where people were declared dead, only to start breathing again. Remember that Californian toddler who was found floating face down in the family pool a couple months ago? They figured she had been in the pool like that for about two hours before they got to her. Well, forty minutes after she was pronounced dead, she started breathing again and responding to touch and sound. Another ten minutes and she would have been placed in a body bag and taken to the morgue.

There was also the case of Gary Dockery, a policeman from Tennessee who woke up seven-and-a-half years after being shot in the head. For all those years he had just lain in a nursing home, sometimes grunting or grimacing, and occasionally blinking his eyes. Then one day he just started talking again, and for about eighteen hours he joked, reminisced, and spoke about the world he left behind back in 1988.

Tom: So, Lou may wake up, is that what you're saying?

Professor Edwards: I have no idea, Tom. We just know that there are times when medical science has to admit that we just don't have all the answers. Now, in the case of the cop who woke up, it's more likely that he was in what is now called a Minimally Responsive State, or MR, and not a true vegetative state. There are only a handful of documented cases of patients awakening from vegetative states after more than a year, and experts concluded that Dockery hadn't been in one.

The distinctions of MR and a truly vegetative state are critical—particularly when some ethicists are urging Americans to sign living wills and encouraging relatives to withhold treatment in cases where recovery seems impossible. Patients who have some awareness are more likely to respond to familiar sights and sounds than those in vegetative states, so their conditions may not be as "hopeless." But determining a patient's status can be difficult. We will just have to wait to find out about Lou.

Tom: So what happened to Gary Dockery?

Professor Edwards: He lived for about one more year. After that day in 1996, he returned to a life of silence although he was more alert than he had been previously.

Tom: I don't mean to sound like Troy, but if he only was awake for one day out of almost eight years, what's the point?

Professor Edwards: First of all, looking at both cases, the fact that the little girl came "back to life" and that Gary Dockery "woke up" shows us that our definitions of consciousness and life are a long way from being precise. When does someone truly die? And, at what level do we continue to experience awareness? The questions are both medical and philosophical. The fact remains that we have really just scratched the surface and often, if not always, the best answer to these questions is that we simply don't know. We can have logical, practical guesses, but we really don't know.

Second, and to Mickey's point, think about the magic of those hours when Dockery could communicate with his family again. Almost eight years after responding to the 911 call that ended with a bullet in his brain, he had another chance to laugh, share feelings, and tell those close to him—including his sons— that he loved them. Was it worth eight years of Twilight-Zone existence for those few bonus hours with his family? My guess is that Gary Dockery would say yes, probably his kids, too. And, let me ask you, Tom, if you knew that you had only eighteen hours to share with your family, what would you tell them and what would you do? Don't answer, just think about it and think about all the men you know who live their entire lives in a kind of Twilight Zone without ever really waking up, not even for a day.

chapter
fourteen

Buy Now...Pay Later
Managing Money and Personal Finances

There was good news about Lou this past week. He is still in a coma, but he is no longer on a respirator. His heart and lungs are operating on their own. His doctor told his mom that a coma rarely lasts more than two to four weeks. He said that Lou was in a "vegetative state," and added that some patients regain a degree of awareness after a vegetative state while others may remain in this state for years or even decades. But we just want to know about Lou, and it's still too soon to tell. Also, the doctor pointed out that the most common complication for a person in a vegetative state is infection such as pneumonia.

This watch-and-wait period is pure agony for Lou's family. The hospital social worker has discussed options that his family is simply not ready to hear—not yet.

Funny how no matter what the situation, we—all of us—seem to quickly move back to our daily routines. Lou is no longer with us and he may never return—we simply don't know. However, life goes on here at Erie. Sales are made, production continues, orders are filled, and paper is processed.

Each day we talk about Lou, shake our heads, laugh as we remember a joke—or rather, laugh as we remember Lou laughing at his own jokes—and feel a personal pain that stays locked up inside. Then we move on to "normal" chatter.

At today's lunch, Troy and Chris present two totally different approaches to personal finance. One is extremely rigid and conservative—the other is frighteningly nonchalant and irresponsible. You guess who matches which description!

Mickey talks about the challenges of money management and the high salaries paid to today's athletes.

"Was that you I saw driving a new Porsche?" I ask Troy.

"All mine, baby, all mine!" says Troy. "Well…mine and the bank's."

"Troy, how can you possibly afford all your toys?" Chris says, in his curiosity. "You have a speed boat, a Harley, a sports car, the finest stereo equipment available, and every gadget in the Sharper Image catalog! Unless you're dealing drugs or have an inheritance stashed away some place, I can't figure out where your money's coming from."

"Leverage, my friend, leverage."

"Leverage?" responds Jim. "What are you talking about?"

"Well, guys," Troy says as he leans forward, "I figure money is cheap these days so I simply use new credit to pay off old bills. I borrow money at a low interest rate to pay off high-interest debt."

"That's fine, Troy," I say, "but that only works if you manage your spending. Consolidating debt is a great idea, but if you keep buying things, you defeat the purpose. Low interest paid on a ton of debt is no different than high interest paid on a small debt."

"Of course there's a difference!" exclaims Troy. "I get to have more toys!"

Laughing, he continues, "You're just jealous, old man, because you got all those kids, and their college expenses are coming up. Plus you got a mortgage and an old lady who won't let you spend a dime without her permission. *And*, she makes you drive a minivan!"

I wince at the minivan comment.

"Seriously," Jim asks, "how many credit cards do you have?"

"Let's see," says Troy, "I've got two VISAs, a MasterCard, an American Express card—that I wouldn't leave home without—one for Best Buy, another for CompUSA, one for Sears, and one for Bacharach where I buy my clothes. Yeah, that's all."

Stunned, all Chris can do is stutter, "What? Are you…? You must be kidding, you're not serious. What?"

"Hold on, Lycra Boy, I almost forgot," Troy says, enjoying Chris's near seizure, complete with sputtered lima beans. "I just got a bunch of blank checks from some bank in California with a note saying I am pre-approved for $10,000 and can start writing checks whenever I want! Pretty cool, huh?"

Flicking one of the errant beans off his shirt, Jim picks up where Chris can't, "What happens when you max out on a card?"

Troy says, without a shred of concern, "I make minimum payments and switch to another card. Hell, if I want, I can always get a brand new card, or transfer a balance from one to another at a better rate and higher limit. Every day I get a new offer in the mail—I even get them in emails."

Regaining his balance, Chris uses his favorite term of endearment, "You idiot," he begins, "all you're doing is guaranteeing a life of debt, poverty, stress, and depression. Even if you paid all your minimums on time, which I highly doubt," (Troy purses his lips, shifts his eyeballs back and forth, and shakes his head), "all you're doing is paying interest while dramatically increasing your principal. As your principal increases, so does your interest payment."

Chris shrieks, his voice rising to a high soprano, "Pretty soon your interest obligations will be higher than your salary!"

"Well, if that happens," says Chris with an indiscernible smile, "I'll just have to hit you up for a loan, old buddy. By the way, what kind of rate are you offering?"

"Troy," Chris says, starting with true concern and civility, "Deborah and I account for every penny we earn and spend. We have a budget and we stick to it."

Sitting up higher on his horse, he continues, "With a house, a child, college loans, and two cars, we still manage to save 30 percent of every dime we earn. We only shop at discount stores, we buy lower grade meat, save coupons, fill-up at the cheapest gas stations, turn the thermostat down in the winter, and *never* use the air conditioning in the summer."

As if there were flags waving and a chorus singing in the background, he continues, "I do our taxes, cut the lawn, repair all of our appliances, and change the oil in my '83 Volvo. We don't need the latest, greatest computer, a big-screen TV, cell phones, a hot tub, vacations to Mexico, or even a weekly night out to a movie and popcorn!"

You can sense the grand finale approaching as he begins to stand up. "We are responsible adults building a future for us and our children. If more people would pay attention to their finances and stop their frivolous spending, we would all be better off. Instead, people like you will go deeper and deeper into debt, stick it to the vendors when you declare bankruptcy, and then do it all over again!

"And who pays? We do. The responsible ones who work, slave, and save so that you can screw us while waving your fancy cars, boats, and toys in our faces!"

"Damn, Broccoli Breath," says Troy, "how can you stand having so much fun? Keep it up and Deborah will take your kid and head off to Austin looking for Ted's wife."

Oh, boy, do I miss Lou now. Certainly he would have stopped the two of them long ago with his wonderful way of diffusing out-of-control tension. I can almost hear him clearing his throat and saying, "Okay, okay, so, listen to this one…."

What Would Mickey Say?
About Managing Money and Personal Finances

Tom: Mickey, you made a ton of money in your day. How did you handle it?

Mickey: It won't come as a shock, I'm sure, when I tell you I was horrible with money and even worse when it came to business contracts. The Yankees once had to bail me out, but finally I got a good lawyer, Roy True, to take care of the Mantle business affairs. Also, let me clear up a myth that some people have about me and money. I never was broke, never went bankrupt, and never lacked for a way to make money. I was just never comfortable around money and left those decisions up to others.

Tom: What do you think about the way in which Chris and Troy deal with their finances?

Mickey: Lord knows I liked a good time, so I can't quite agree with Chris, although I sure do respect his will power. Troy just flat out scares me. I never could stand the idea of being in debt. I once had a chance to invest in a real estate deal that gave a great tax write-off. All I had to do was put up a little cash and sign a note with some other fellows for about $300,000. My lawyer checked it out and said it was fine—there was a zero chance that I would have to pay it off. Well, after a few nights of tossing and turning and worrying about the money, I had Roy get me out of the deal. I just couldn't sleep knowing that I owed somebody money. What Troy is doing is crazy.

Tom: Why do you think you were so cautious?

Mickey: It must be because I grew up so poor back in Commerce and how dead set against borrowing my dad was. I bet we were the only family in Commerce that paid cash for our groceries—everyone else bought their groceries on credit. In fact, the grocer was so pleased with dad that he let us kids pick out a free bag of candy every once in while. Maybe that's why I stayed away from debt—I got free candy!

Tom: But you had some pretty good business deals along the way, didn't you?

Mickey: I had some good ones, like Mickey Mantle's Restaurant in New York City, but some of 'em weren't too good. Let me tell you a story I told in Cooperstown when I was inducted into the Baseball Hall of Fame.

In 1957, Harold Youngman built a Holiday Inn in Joplin, Missouri, and called it Mickey Mantle's Holiday Inn. I was a partner and we were doin' pretty good there. Mr. Youngman said, 'You know, you're half of this thing, so why don't you do something for it?' We had real good chicken there and I made up this slogan: 'To get a better piece of chicken, you'd have to be a rooster.' And I don't know if that's what closed up our Holiday Inn or not, but we didn't do too good after that. No, actually, it was really a good deal, but I just love to tell that story.

Tom: Any advice?

Mickey: The only advice I have is, don't be like Troy! And, if you're fortunate enough to make some extra money, find someone like I did to help tell you what to do with it. But, check the guy out before you give him your money.

The Professor Speaks
About Managing Money and Personal Finances

Tom: Any thing to say about finances, Professor?

Professor Edwards: I'll come back to Chris in a moment, but let's go after the obvious concern that Troy presents. First of all, he reminds me of the Ogden Nash quote, "Some debts are fun when you are acquiring them, but none are fun when you set about retiring them." Let's take a look at Troy and use him to create the Five Warning Signs of Dollar Danger. You know you're in a fiscal pickle when…

1) *You use one credit card to pay off another.* Clear danger when this happens. Don't kid yourself into believing that all you need is a better interest rate and all will be well. Your problem concerns buying habits, not bill-paying habits. People who pay their credit card debt with another credit card are the same folks who choose one store in a mall over another based upon which credit card they think is closer to the max (they don't want to be embarrassed).

2) *All you pay is interest.* Credit card companies are more than willing to bump up your credit ceiling as long as you pay your interest. Like Chris told Troy, the danger here is that before long, all you can pay is the interest—you have no money available for the principal.

3) *You have more than three credit cards in your wallet.* One credit card is all you should ever need. However, let's be liberal and allow for a general credit card like a VISA or MasterCard, a favorite department store card (after all, they gave you a 15 percent discount off your first purchase), and a separate VISA, MasterCard, or American Express card for legitimate business expenses. Any more cards than three and you are headed for trouble. More than likely, if this is you, you already know this.

4) *Your "wants" dwarf your "needs."* New cars, designer clothes, the latest gadgets, trips to sunny places, and fine art all add a certain spice to life, but if you can barely afford the main meal it's best to go lightly with the spice. Besides, after awhile all those things simply contribute to more and more stress in your life, particularly if you have champagne taste and a beer budget. I believe it was the philosopher, Mick Jagger, who once screeched, "You can't always get what you want, but if you try sometime, you just might find, you get what you need."

5) *You don't think this section has anything to do with you.* Careful, the Fiscal Pickle sneaks up on the unsuspecting. If something compelled you to read this far, you probably already need watch out for the first four danger signs.

Tom: So, how do you avoid becoming a "Troy"?

Professor Edwards: Other than the obvious counters to the above, here are five things you can do:

1) *Decide what you need to make you comfortable.* Learn to distinguish between your "wants" and your "needs." Being as strict as Chris takes all the fun out of life. Everyone should have a few things that they just love, even if they are not practical. Just try and develop simple tastes!

2) *If you can't pay your bills, ask for help immediately.* Young people in particular don't seem to understand what credit history is. When you are late with payments, or worse, just quit making payments, this information is recorded and contributes to your credit rating. This tells future lenders, like a bank or a mortgage company, what kind of a risk you are. Not only does it impact whether or not you can borrow money, it deter-

mines what rate you will pay—the better the risk, the lower the interest rate. If you are going to be late, make a call and talk to someone. If you simply can't afford the current terms, tell them. It's in the best interest of the lenders to keep their customers happy. If brought into the loop early enough, most creditors will work with you to set up a payment schedule you can afford *without hurting your credit rating.*

3) *Cash is king.* This is an old saying and for good reason. In some cases, retailers will provide a discount when paying with cash. Another reason is that when you pay with cash, you actually *see* the dollars slip from your hands into another's. This can be very sobering and turn an impulse purchase into a reflective, maybe for another time.

4) *Use a debit card.* Almost as good as cash, this way of paying requires that you already have the money in the bank. This minimizes or eliminates overspending, interest payments, and buyer's remorse. Of course, it does only minor good if you forget to write the purchase down and don't deduct it from your checkbook.

5) *Beware of ATMs.* Remember when you were little and your mom or dad would say to you, "Child, do you think money grows on trees?" Well, of course, the answer today would be, "Nope, it comes out of the ATM!" Crisp five, ten, or twenty dollar bills that zip out of a machine on your demand make impulse buying almost as easy as credit cards. Yes, the good part is that you must have the money in to take it out, but the danger comes when you can find an ATM on any street corner, any bar, in all the shopping malls, and almost anywhere in the world. At the very least, only take out the money you expect to spend on that particular trip. The more you have to dig for the card, the more you will have to think about what you are doing.

chapter

fifteen

Bottom of the Ninth
Taking Stock, Licking Wounds, Celebrating Victories, and Planning for Another Year

Nobody loves life like him who is growing old.
— Sophocles

How old would you be if you didn't know how old you was?
— Satchel Paige

*P*layed the final game of the season last night. This past two weeks without Lou on the field were very strange. There's still no change in his condition.

Surprisingly, we won both games, but honestly there was little satisfaction in either victory. Not that we didn't enjoy playing. In fact, it seemed to help everyone's mood. Baseball and softball have always done that for me—gotten my mind off of daily stressors or life problems. Didn't really matter if I was playing or just watching.

In spite of all the bickering and squabbling during the past three months, I have to say that I enjoy seeing these guys Thursday nights and Fridays for lunch. I will miss the season. While perhaps crude and seemingly tactless, these guys are refreshing. Each of them tends to say what's on his mind—not a whole lot of mystery or ambiguity. And, as for the barbs and cheap shots, it's like going to a hockey game and watching a fight. The same guys who drop their gloves are likely to be hoisting a few cold ones together after the game.

At lunch today, we talk about things that happened both on and off the field. Or, rather, Jim talks and we listen. Jim has reached out more and more since he started therapy. Today, he dominates the conversation and forces all of us to think about our futures.

In spite of Jim taking direct aim at Troy, there is an atmosphere of affection and even respect hanging over the table. The affection remains unspoken, of course—but it is clearly present.

Mickey becomes very philosophical as he presents a quick snapshot of his life, complete with joys and disappointments. He talks about the lessons learned from his time at the Betty Ford Center and gives parting advice for anyone who will listen.

The professor offers key advice about living a good life without causing harm to others, and about taking accountability for your actions.

Limping to the table (pulled the same muscle I did earlier in the season), I see that Troy, Chris, and Jim are in an animated discussion. It's nice to see that Jim is the one who is most animated. Last week, he confided in me that he is seeing a therapist and is feeling better and stronger. It shows!

"One of my favorite Yogi quotes," says Jim as I sit down, "is when he said, 'If I didn't wake up I'd still be sleeping.' That's how I feel about what's happened these last few months. If I didn't wake up I'd still be sleeping, or maybe worse."

Troy looks at him with a twist of his head and a scrunched-up face, "What does that mean?"

"It means," answers Chris, "that a whole lot of men walk around conscious but not necessarily awake." He adds with a surprising smile and a pleasant wink, "That shouldn't be too difficult for you to understand."

"That's exactly what it means," says Jim with enthusiasm. "I am now awake—or, at least, I'm awakening. And, a lot of credit goes to you guys."

"Well, you're welcome," says Troy. "Now, as Lou would say, 'Pass the salt.'"

"What do mean by that, Jim," I ask. "How did we help? What did we do?"

"It really isn't what you did, exactly. It's more the things you guys said and what happened around here over the past few months," answers Jim.

"Certainly nothing that Lycra Boy could have said," replies Troy. "He just thinks he knows everything. Ain't that right, Doc?"

"Not today, pee-brain, not today. I'm in too good a mood to be offended by mental midgets. I ran a personal best, 5:22-mile, this morning," Chris says, with a puff of his chest. "Or to put it in terms you would understand, Troy-Boy, I ran a mile in the time it takes you to smoke a joint."

"You must be mistaking my smoking a joint with how long it takes you to make love to your wife," Troy shoots back.

Oh Lou, Oh Lou, Oh Lou, I think. Where are you, Lou?

I take a deep breath and jump in. "Speaking of making love..." I begin, as all heads turn and give me a strange inquisitive look that says, McGregor? A joke?

"Did you guys know that bankers do it with interest, detectives do it under cover, gardeners do it in the bushes, DJs do it on request, and Frank Sinatra did it his way?"

Nothing. Nada. Zilch. Zero. All I can imagine is the sound of a distant drummer's rim shot and an old comedian tapping the microphone and asking, "Hello? Hello? Is this thing on?"

Finally, painfully, and oh, so politely, Chris says, "No, Tom, I didn't know that."

Oh Lou, Oh Lou, Oh Lou, I think, again. Where are you, Lou?

Ignoring Beavis, Butthead, and the tired, balding comedian from the Catskills, Jim continues. "Think back on the last three months and all the things that have happened, just with people here at this table.

"We have dealt with some pretty heavy things—Harvey's death, Lou's coma, Troy getting arrested, and Ted leaving. We've also insulted each other, shared personal stuff, and laughed at Lou's stupid jokes."

Wow, none of us have really seen the philosopher side of Jim, so we're intrigued and somewhat surprised as we give him our undivided attention.

"Yeah," says Chris, "but how has that awakened you?"

"Well, while I didn't want to talk much about it at first, things have been kind of difficult at home. Not always, really, just the past year or so. However, the worse they became, the more I pulled away." He looks down at his tray and then back to each of us. "I got so I was living in my own little world, and it was pretty dark. In fact, it was more like a cave. It was a place to hide from Shelley's drugs, Mildred's menopause, my depression about getting older, and Lucille's illness.

"You see, from the time I was a kid, I would run away from my problems by shooting baskets by myself at the neighborhood school or reading science fiction magazines like *Fantasy* or *Science Fiction Digest*. Anything, just so I wouldn't have to think about any problems at home. I just wanted to escape. I continued to do that as an adult.

"At any rate," he continues, "it just seemed easier to ignore my problems and pretend that things were just fine—ignore my pain and fear. And it worked—or at least I thought it did until everything came crashing down this year."

Troy looks like he's about to say something until Chris shoots him a look.

"Sorry for the Jerry Springer confession, guys," says Jim, picking up on Troy's growing unease. "But my shrink says it's good for me, and besides, I think you may feel the same way about some of this stuff."

Troy can't hold back, "Damn, Jim," he says giving Chris a "screw-you" look. "No offense, but way too much information, man. Can't you just cut to the chase? What woke you up?"

"Actually, Troy," Jim says, not seeming the least bit annoyed by Troy's rudeness. "you're a big part of what did it—what woke me up."

"Me? What did I do?"

With a hesitant look Jim begins. "Troy, you're a smart guy with a lot going for you. But, you're also a time bomb with a fast clock," he says, as he eases into a comfortable tone.

"A few weeks ago, after Spatalie's suicide, someone, probably Chris," he motions at Iverson, "said something about there being a number of ways to commit suicide."

Now, looking straight at Troy, Jim continues, "He was talking about Lou and his diet, smokes, and beer, but his comment made me think of you, Troy, not Lou."

"You're a bright, young kid who's pissing his life away. You're constantly flirting with disaster and you think it's funny." He pauses, looks down, and then directly into Troy's eyes. "Troy, you're one continuous side-show of drugs, booze, fights, meaningless sex, fast cars, and irresponsible spending. I'm sorry if you don't want to hear this," he says, beginning to slow down, "but it's true.

"I like you. You've got good looks, charm, charisma, and, in many ways, you remind me of me, when I was your age." Jim sits back in his chair. "You put up a big front of not caring, and you say some pretty shocking things, but my sense is that you're a decent young man who's pretty damn scared deep inside just like I was. So scared, that you figure it's easier to pretend you don't care than it is to open your heart."

Troy starts to speak, but Jim holds up his hand and continues, "At first, when all my problems were heating up at home, I envied your youth, freedom, and give-a-rip attitude. Then you started to anger me. I felt you were just a spoiled brat with no sense of responsibility and a hard-on for the whole world."

He looks around the table and you can tell that nothing is going to stop him—not now. Troy is listening. "Then, when you told us about your dad leaving your mom, I realized that it wasn't you that pissed me off, it was the fact that I saw me in you! I was the one who was filled with anger, hatred, and bitterness. I have been since I was your age, even younger. And it was me who was flirting with the idea of suicide. You see, my dad also left us. He abandoned us—abandoned me. But he didn't do it with a woman—he did it with a gun to his head, just like Spatalie.

"Troy, besides associating my youth with yours, that story you told about your dad leaving helped me to understand why I've been so angry, so depressed, and feeling so alone. You see, my dad killed himself when I was fifteen. That was about the same time I started hiding in science fiction books and escaping from the world with sports. Up until that time, I was happy, a good student, and the best jock on the block. Life was good and the future was even better. Everything changed after that summer. Everything. Mom left us—she didn't die or run off with the milkman—she just wasn't there, anymore. I couldn't play high school sports because I had to work. Because I was the oldest, I felt a responsibility to take care of my brother and sister."

He continues, "You started me thinking about all of this, but it was Chris and Lou who brought it all to a head. Chris?" Jim says, looking past Troy. "Remember that day when I got so ticked off at you, that I left the table?" he asks. "Remember?" Chris nods.

"Well, I was angry because you were right when you said that part of Shelley's problem was me. You were 100 percent on target, I just didn't want to hear it."

"Oh, please," says Troy. "Don't tell him he's right. He really doesn't need encouragement." We all laugh.

"And Lou...," Jim continues, "thinking about Lou and what happened to him has given me a new appreciation for life. After seeing him lying in that bed, I realized that I didn't want to die. In fact, better than that, I knew then that I wanted to live!"

On a roll, he looks at me. "Tommy? Remember when you were talking about you and Laurie and how menopause messed up your marriage?"

"Well," I say, "it really was Laurie and me that almost messed up our marriage, but, yes, I remember. Laurie still gets tears in her eyes when she thinks of those days. She honestly thinks that without the hormone replacements, she would have gone nuts and our marriage would have collapsed. Don't forget, I was just as wacky as she was, and it took honest communication as much as chemistry to get us back on the right track."

"Right," responds Jim. "I told Millie and she's now taking some kind of natural estrogen supplements that make her feel much better. We also agreed to go to family counseling for Shelley's drug problem, and from there I went into my own counseling." Jim is now beaming. "Don't know where all this is going, but it sure feels better than it did a few months ago.

"So, you see. You guys have helped me to wake up. Now that I'm awake, I have a couple of choices. I can move forward with my life trying to make it better, or I can hit the snooze button, like my buddy, Troy," he says, with a wink toward our young friend.

"Like I said before," says Troy with a sincere smile, "you're welcome. Now, will you please shut up and pass the salt?"

We all smile. Something's changed, or is changing—I'm not sure exactly what, but it feels right. Already I'm looking forward to next year's softball season.

What Would Mickey Say?
About the Bottom of the Ninth

Tom: Well, Mick, any wrap-up reflections on the season?

Mickey: I can't help but continue to wish I had another shot at all of this. Another chance to make different decisions, to appreciate what I had, and to contribute more. I guess there's a reason for everything, including all the mistakes I made, but it's hard when you start to know better and think about what you should have done.

Tom: Clearly you made mistakes, but to your credit you recognized them and tried to set them straight before you died. You also did many things right in your life. If you were to honor Mickey Mantle, to give your own eulogy, what would you say?

Mickey: Oh man, that's a tough one, Tom. I'm not that good with words and I wasn't brought up to brag or talk a whole lot about myself.

Tom: Don't think of it like that. Speak like a fan of Mickey Mantle's or, better than that, someone who just watched and followed Mickey's life objectively. What would that person say about the positive things you left behind?

Mickey: Well, let's see how it goes. I guess I'd like to say that I did the right thing when I told the kids out there not to be like me. I mean, not to do the wrong things I did. I want the kids to have fun and play to win and I want them to take care of themselves, treat others nice, and respect their parents and teachers.

Tom: You're getting the idea. But try to put it into a eulogy or a testimonial, like a dinner speech honoring Mickey Mantle.

Mickey: Kind of like Bob Costas?

Tom: Yes, just like that. Like the eulogy Costas gave at your funeral.

Mickey: Nope—can't do it. I'm just not that comfortable talking about myself like that. But how about if I just tell you what I liked about the eulogy— what parts meant the most to me?

Tom: Fair enough.

Mickey: I liked the teammate part right at the beginning. I always thought about the game as a team sport. It burns me when I think of some of today's players who just think about themselves and how much more money they can make. The reason I always kept my head down when I ran the bases after a home run was because I didn't want to show up the pitcher, you know, rub it in. I didn't want to make the game about me. The records were nice and everything, but in the end it was about the team winning.

I also like the fact that fans felt that in some way I represented them. Because that's how I felt. That's also part of the reason I would kick a water cooler or toss a helmet now and then. I was angry at myself when I didn't do well, but, also, I didn't want to disappoint the fans. They paid good money to come and watch us play and my job was to give the guy in the bleachers his money's worth.

Tom: How did it make you feel knowing that guys in their forties and fifties continued to think of you as their hero long after they were kids?

Mickey: Boy, I never quite got that one, but I learned to accept it and was glad that I somehow touched their lives in a good way. I played most of my best baseball after WWII, just about the time that television was taking off. I guess people thought of me as representing what this country was all about. Of course, Dizzy Dean and Pee Wee Reese kinda helped spread that image with their Saturday Game of the Week, and Mel Allen, Voice of the Yankees, talked it up pretty good, too. Yeah, I'm glad people enjoyed what I did. But, you know, it kinda made me feel bad knowing that I could have done better. There were plenty of other guys playing ball in those years that deserved the respect and affection more than me. There was Ted Williams, Stan Musial, Willie Mays, Al Kaline, Warren Spahn, and, of course, Jackie Robinson, Hank Aaron, and Roy Campenella. All those guys deserved it more than me.

Tom: Then why you, Mick? Why you?

Mickey: Oh, I don't know. I think they liked the long home runs—everyone does. I do, too. Also, maybe because they knew I always gave my best on the field, even when I was hurt pretty bad. I didn't whine much. I also enjoyed myself out there and I think people liked that. I had a good time playing baseball and maybe it reminded guys of when they were kids, just enjoying a game. The fact that I was from Oklahoma, just like Will Rogers, might have helped, too. I sure wasn't very slick when I showed up in New York City. I was just a kid from the sticks who loved to play baseball like millions of other kids from small towns all over the country. Maybe that was part of it. I wasn't real flashy and I was kind of a bumpkin—you know, shy and a little bashful.

Tom: What are you most proud of?

Mickey: The way our family came together toward the end. I think that's what it's all about—family and forgiveness. I'm real happy about that. I just wish it had happened earlier. The organ donor program is another thing I'm real pleased about. I know it was controversial, me receiving the liver and all, but the publicity helped thousands of others and had a big impact on organ donations. I'm pretty proud of that.

Tom: Any final words for our friends here—our lunchroom gang?

Mickey: I pretty much said all I have to say about what these guys talked about this season. I want Troy to listen hard to what Jim just told him. That took a lot of guts and caring on Jim's part. I wish more people had spoken to me like that when I was Troy's age. I know it's hard when you're in your twenties to ever think you could end up like I did, but if guys like Troy would just pause for a second and think about possible consequences, they would be so much better off. Troy's got a shot at making it if he just survives the next several years, or however long it takes for him to grow up. Problem today is that there are so many ways to screw yourself up, and that kid seems to know how to find most of them.

Tom: How about Chris and Jim?

Mickey: Oh man, Chris needs to lighten up! He's got a lot of book sense, but his people skills stink. Nobody likes a goody-goody and a know-it-all. Until Chris gets off his high horse and learns a little humility, he will turn off a lot of people who really need to hear what he has to say.

Jim is on the right track. In fact, Jim is the real bright light here. He got some help and is taking steps to move himself and his family forward. I thought we lost him when that Spatalie guy killed himself. He could have gone either way. I understand what it's like to be in that position. I never felt better or worse than when I went to the Betty Ford Clinic. There were days when I didn't know if I was going to make it. But I stuck with it. Sounds like Jim's buying into the pain and hard work it will take to keep him moving on down the road. It will pay off. Jim's a good one. I hope he continues to bug Troy, too. He just may turn out to be the father neither one of them had.

Tom: How about Ted Johnson?

Mickey: You know, in every bunch there's always one that gets away. He's the one. My advice would be for others to stay clear of that guy. I'm sorry. I sincerely hope he turns it around, but from where I stand, he just never got it. Maybe he never will. Life is short and if I get to make out the guest list, that guy ain't coming to the party. The problem is that he is real smart, good looking, and quite the talker. All great things for a sales guy. Trouble is that what he's selling is poison and he doesn't care who buys as long as he gets what he wants. Here's my advice—unless you're a social worker, or maybe his mama—run and don't look back. His wife and kids are better off without him.

Tom: Mickey, what about Lou? Assuming he comes out of this, what good words do you have for him?

Mickey: Lou makes me feel real bad. Of course I hope he pulls through, and when he does, my guess is that he will make some serious changes in the way he lives his life. It's just too bad that something like this has to happen before guys like Lou get it.

It's like when you asked me if I had any advice for the young Mickey Charles Mantle. Yeah, sure, I had all kinds of advice, but I doubted that he would listen. Someone once said that a blind man doesn't know he's walking toward the edge until after he takes his last step. Let's hope that something breaks Lou's fall and he gets to climb back up on the road and can try this thing again. This time without the blindfold.

Tom: And last, but I hope not least, how about me, Mick. Any advice?

Mickey: I don't like giving all this advice, Tom, but I just hope you realize how good you got it. Sounds like you had quite a scare with your marriage, but you and your wife were able to pull it together before you lost each other. I'm real glad that you did—for you and your family.

Also, treasure those kids of yours. Give them all the good stuff in life. You know, the kind of stuff you can't charge on a credit card. Hugs, and time, and lots and lots of love. Play with them, listen to them, and don't be afraid to tell them when they are wrong, even if it means they will be mad at you for doing it. Also, be an example for your kids—not just in how to do things right, but how to fix things when you screw up. We all screw up, but not very many guys know how to fix things when they do. I guess maybe that's why they drink, do drugs, or even leave when the road gets rough. They don't know what to do, so they just figure out a way to escape so they don't have to think about it. I know I did.

Hey, and Tom, at some point, give it up, guy. Sure, keep playing softball, skiing, bowling or whatever activity you enjoy, but get it out of your head that you are still twenty! You're not, and all the ACE bandages and ointment in the world won't give you back your youth. No reason not to stay active all your life, just pay attention and take better care of that body of yours.

Tom: Anything more for any of us?

Mickey: Nope. Just be nice to others, always do your best, and enjoy the life you've got. And, of course, don't be like me. That's about it. Pretty simple stuff. Like Yogi says, "Give 100 percent in the first half of the game, and if that isn't enough, in the second half you give what's left."

The Professor Speaks
About the Bottom of the Ninth

Tom: What would you like to say as we wrap up the season, Professor Edwards?

Professor Edwards: Oh, Tom, there are so many, many lessons here. If I may borrow a line from Yogi, "You can observe a lot just by watching." And, I might add, you can also hear if you listen, as well.

The overriding message from Mickey is for all of us to embrace the gifts we've been given and to take responsibility for our actions. Certainly, there is also the plea to wake up and take control of our lives now, while we can truly make a difference, and not wait until some horrific event reminds us of our mortality and shakes us into action.

In the fall of 2003, Darryl Strawberry, an eight-time All-Star who overcame drug addiction, prison, and cancer, was hired as a player development instructor for the Yankees. "I want to be a positive role model for somebody," Strawberry said in an interview. "I didn't reach my full potential. Hopefully, I can help somebody reach theirs."

Mickey couldn't have said it any better.

Tom: But to your point, Professor, do men have to have some catastrophic event to shake them from a hurtful and self-destructive path? And, more importantly, how do they keep from going down that path to begin with? Stories like Mickey's and Darryl Strawberry's are inspirational and show that guys can pull it out in the bottom of the ninth, so to speak, but the Prodigal Son story is getting somewhat old. For some of us it almost suggests that all is well as long as you wake up at the end and apologize for all the hurtful, harmful, and just plain stupid things you did in your life.

Professor Edwards: A sincere apology supported by action is very powerful and needs to be respected. Of course, the emphasis here is on the word, "sincere." We all make mistakes; however, the key is what follows the words—what we do when we realize we have harmed others and ourselves. An apology without change is fraudulent, dangerous, and cruel.

No doubt, Mickey offered up many apologies along the way. The problem was that, like too many of us, he was let off the hook too easily. No one ever really called him to task for his boorish behavior. He was allowed and even encouraged to brush aside his wrongdoings as long as he continued to be Mickey Mantle. It goes for Darryl Strawberry, Robert Downey, Jr., Michael Jackson, Russell Crowe, Mike Tyson, Bill Clinton, and dozens of others.

Fortunately, most men don't have to wait until the brink of death, public humiliation, or financial ruin before they wake up. The vast majority of guys walk, stumble, and adjust as they move through life gaining wisdom, strength, and perspective as they move from one stage to the next. This occurs, in part, because someone—actually several people—helped keep the boys and men in their life from straying too far before being challenged to account for their behavior.

Bottom line advice is pretty much what Mickey said: guys need to pay attention, do their best, treat others fairly, and enjoy the journey. Oh, and most important, be accountable and responsible for your actions. No more whining, complaining, and pointing fingers at others. In other words, be a man, be a real man!

Tom: See ya next season, Professor?

Professor Edwards: You bet, Tom, you bet.

endnotes

[1] Bobby Richardson was the starter at second base for the great New York Yankee teams that won five consecutive pennants and two World Series from 1960 through 1964. Bobby retired at the age of thirty-one to devote himself to his family and interests including a run for Congress and work with the Fellowship of Christian Athletes.

[2] Billy Martin, five-time manager of the New York Yankees, won two pennants and one World Series (1977); he also managed Minnesota, Detroit, Texas, and Oakland, and played on five Yankee world champions with Mickey in the 1950s.

[3] Whitey Ford, all-time leader in World Series wins (10); led AL in wins three times; won Cy Young and World Series MVP in 1961 with the New York Yankees; 236–106 record.

[4] Casey Stengel, Hall of Fame manger guided the New York Yankees to ten AL pennants and seven World Series titles from 1949–60.

[5] Mickey married Merlyn Johnson on December 23, 1952. He was twenty years old. They were married for forty-three years.

[6] Yogi Berra, the Yankee catcher, and his wife Carmen. Yogi was elected to the Baseball Hall of Fame in 1972.

[7] Clete Boyer was another steady Yankee who played with Mickey from 1959–66.

[8] Hodgkin's Disease skipped Mickey and killed his son, Billy, in 1994.

[9] Billy Martin died in a single-car accident on Christmas Day, 1989.

[10] On January 7, 1994, Mickey entered the Betty Ford Clinic for a thirty-two-day stay. He never drank again. Not even two months later when on March 12, 1994, his son Billy died from Hodgkin's Disease at the age of thirty-six.

[11] Ralph Houk coached the Yankees from 1961–63 and again from 1966–73.

[12] Hank Bauer played with Mickey on the Yankees from 1951–59.

[13] Brooks Robinson played with Baltimore from 1955–77 and entered the Hall of Fame in 1983.

[14] NOTE: Our fictitious Professor Edwards is a blend of my thirty years in the field of health promotion, today's research, professional observations, and personal opinion. Information is pulled from the fields of medicine, law, and human behavior.

[15] Sports Illustrated, "Over the Edge", Yeager, D., Bamberger, M, Vol. 86, Issue 15, April 14, 1997.

[16]
$$BMI = \frac{weight\ (pounds) \times 705}{height\ (inches)^2}$$

about the
author

Currently, Michael serves as Executive Lead, Health & Wellness Initiative, Blue Cross Blue Shield of Rhode Island. Prior to this engagement, Michael served as the Chairman of The National Center for Health Promotion, a health and productivity consulting organization he co-founded in 1977.

Michael is widely published and is a frequent director, consultant, and advisor to numerous prestigious boards and organizations including The Men's Health Network, The Lance Armstrong Foundation, and The Department of Defense. In addition, he has written and contributed to corporate policies for several major US corporations.

A graduate of the University of Michigan with an MA degree in Education, he is a frequent guest lecturer for a number of UM departments. Michael has appeared on over 200 television and radio stations throughout North America and has been interviewed by numerous print publications including *Newsweek*, *USA Today*, and *The Wall Street Journal*. His work in the area of behavior change and healthcare consumer advocacy has been featured on the ABC News program, *20/20*, *The CBS Morning Show*, CNN, and MSNBC. Michael serves on a number of national cancer boards and, at the request of former President George H. W. Bush, is a member of C-Change, which is comprised of the nation's key cancer leaders from government, business, and nonprofit sectors.

Michael is the author of *Voices from the Edge: Life Lessons from the Cancer Community*, *Moments...Not Years*, *Relaxation*, and *Marketing Healthy Lifestyles: Advancing Health Promotion as a Profit Center and Cost Containment Strategy*.

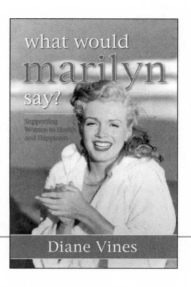

**If you enjoyed *What Would Mickey Say?* check out
*What Would Marilyn Say? Supporting Women to Health
and Happiness* by Diane Vines.
Buy a copy for the woman in your life—or several
copies for all the women in your life.**

Similar in content to the Mickey Mantle book, *What Would Marilyn
Say?* deals with women's health as seen through the eyes of a fictional
group of women who are returning to college. These women meet weekly
to discuss their lives, health, and happiness. Overseeing the group is a
virtual professor and Marilyn Monroe, who comments on what she would
have done differently about her health had she survived that fateful night
in 1962. *What Would Marilyn Say?* also reveals the truth behind the iconic
image of the starlet whose perfect facade masked a dark inner turmoil.

Available online at arnicapublishing.com!